Super Nutrition for Men

# Super Nutrition for Men

### And the Women Who Love Them

## Ann Louise Gittleman, M.S.
### Certified Nutrition Specialist

#### with Susan Stockton, M.A.

M. Evans and Company, Inc.
New York

M. Evans and Company, Inc.
216 East 49th Street
New York, NY 10017


Library of Congress Cataloging-in-Publication Data
CIP Data is available from the Library of Congress.

Text design by Charles de Kay

Manufactured in the United States of America

First Edition

9  8  7  6  5  4  3  2

**Dedication**

*This book is lovingly dedicated to
Arthur Gittleman, my father—
the first man in my life.*

# ACKNOWLEDGMENTS

First and foremost my greatest thanks to Susan Stockton, my right hand, and to Carol Faye Templeton, my brilliant, little computer whiz.

I also owe a lot to the men in my life.

There have been many male role models whom I have learned from since I was a little girl including my father and my brother, Stuart. And so what better way to recognize them than in a book dedicated to the good health and longevity of men:

To Aaron Kriwitsky—my grandfather—a religious scholar who taught me the holiness of the written and spoken word.

To Rabbi Haskel Lindenthal—my religious school mentor—who cultivated in me the value of learning and study.

To Emerich Ohlbaum—one of my Dad's closest friends—whose amazing work ethic and lively personality never ceased to amaze me.

To John Harris—my high school English teacher—whose voice I still hear in my head as I compose my manuscripts.

To Edward Aldworth—a truly elegant gentleman who is both kind and shrewd.

To Chuck Kambourian—the most talented and devoted family man I know.

To Don Meredith—a living legend who is as charming in real life as he was on Monday night football.

To Chuck Diker—a great business leader and humanitarian.

To Jeff Howard—a man whose integrity and forward thinking I greatly admire.

To John Desgrey—a man who taught me how to visualize and make dreams come true.

And to the other great guys who have contributed to my life in their own way. Here's to Josh Rubenstein, my childhood dear friend who went on to become a writer and spokesperson for the political prisoners of the world; to Paul Kimatian, a talented producer who taught me "how to do lunch" and guided me during my years in California; and to James William Templeton who has made my life complete.

# Contents

# CHAPTER 1

# WHY A NUTRITION BOOK FOR MEN?

Like winning the lottery, this book will change the way you live your life. If you're tired of the same old diet and exercise programs that just don't work, and if you can use some practical advice on sex, fitness, substance abuse, and how to protect your heart and prostate naturally, then this book is for you. *Super Nutrition for Men*, based on cutting-edge research and my own clinical experience over twenty years, is for everyone from eighteen to eighty.

You will discover how cutting down on carbs and upping the right fats will turn your body into a fat-burning machine. You'll learn about the latest wave in getting fit fast—the 40/30/30 plan—used by world-class athletes to significantly improve athletic performance and recovery. The good news about the 40/30/30 plan is that it allows even the couch potato to access stored body fat for fuel. This plan helps increase energy, improve concentration and attention span, increase lean muscle mass, and curb food cravings.

You'll begin to look at food from a whole new perspective—as fuel for both the body and the mind. You'll be introduced to the concept of the hormonal impact of food and its power to impact peak performance, mood, and overall health.

Many innovative programs for protecting the prostate, healing the heart, super charging sex, controlling hair loss, overcoming addictions, and eating at home and on the go are outlined in these pages. All of these programs can fit into busy schedules. Most of them require minor

1

adjustments in the way you live. Others may not be quite as simple, but the rewards will be worth it.

*Super Nutrition for Men* is a no-nonsense handbook that contains answers to questions most frequently asked by my male clients:

Is it really possible to avoid prostate problems?
Can I still eat healthy if I'm a meat and potatoes man?
Is there anything I can do about my thinning hair?
If heart disease runs in the family, are there natural therapies I can
   use to prevent it?
Any sexual secrets I should know?
What is the latest on drugless treatments to get off caffeine? Nicotine?
   Marijuana? Cocaine?

This book is unique, different than anything you've ever read before on men's health. Just turn to the chapter on "Super Nutrition for Substance Abuse" and you'll see what I mean. The programs I suggest are derived from the research of some of the most respected authorities around the world.

Knowledge is power. Staying in optimum shape and achieving great overall health takes know-how. You will learn all the formulas to staying on top, formulas which you haven't read about in any other books, magazine articles, or seen on TV.

You will find up-to-the-minute health and nutrition strategies all throughout *Super Nutrition for Men*. And, by the way, this book is not just for men. It's for the women who love them. So, don't be afraid to have your wife, girlfriend, or significant other peruse these pages with you. Or, better still, get her her own copy.

Now, let's shift gears a bit.

## WHERE MEN STAND

Here are the real life, hardcore statistics and data that compelled me to write *Super Nutrition for Men*. Men lead in eight of the ten top causes of death in the U.S. Men are reluctant to seek medical care. When they finally do decide to see a physician, their illnesses have progressed to a more critical state. Men are equally reluctant to seek counseling and emotional support and constitute only 30 percent of the patients who consult psychologists and psychiatrists: This despite the fact that men abuse alcohol and drugs three times as much as women do, commit over 90 percent of violent crime, and kill themselves three times as often.

Although heart disease remains the number one killer among men, only one-third of those in the forty-five to sixty-four age group have ever had their cholesterol level checked. Among men over fifty, only one out of two knows the warning signs of prostate or colorectal cancer, and one out of five reports being too embarrassed to discuss the matter with their doctor. A mere 22 percent of men over forty report having had a digital rectal exam to check for prostate problems in the previous year, despite the fact that annual DRE exams are recommended by authorities for middle-aged men.

While men are far less likely to go on diets or join weight-loss programs, they're no less likely to **be** overweight. In fact, statistics reveal that more American men are obese than are American women (26.1 percent compared to 25.1 percent). Maybe this has something to do with the fact that only 47 percent of men pay attention to food's nutritional content.

Male pattern obesity (where weight is concentrated in the middle of the body) is more dangerous than the female pattern (more weight in the thighs and hips), for it increases the risk of developing cardiovascular disease. Obesity is also a risk factor for diabetes and is linked to the development of hypertension, stroke, gall bladder disease, sleep apnea, musculoskeletal problems, and certain forms of cancer. The cold, hard, bottom line according to Dr. Morton Shaevitz, Director of Eating Disorders Programs at Scripps Clinic and Research Foundation, is that "fat men die young."

And yet, men lose weight more easily than women for reasons that are largely physiological. While men are less likely to take overt steps to control their weight, evidence is strong that they care about their appearance. A growing number are choosing to have aesthetic (or plastic) surgery. Over the past twenty-five years, 30 percent of such surgeries have been performed on men. Procedures commonly sought by men include liposuction, eyelid surgery, rhinoplasties (nose jobs), and face lifts.

The good news is that losing weight and keeping it off will increase longevity. In fact, losing only 10 percent or less of body weight can increase life span, as well as substantially improve hypertension, adult onset diabetes, and cardiovascular disease. Men may dislike the idea of dieting, but they're good at losing weight when they resolve to do so and take the appropriate steps.

## STRESS

One of the biggest problems with the Standard American Diet (SAD) is that it stresses the body. It acts as a stressor because it depletes nutrient reserves which in turn decreases the body's ability to handle stress. This is a special problem for men, who are more susceptible to stress-related disorders, due to their tendency to:

deny problems rather than deal with them
hold feelings in
be reluctant to admit setbacks

These factors contribute to increased rates of heart attacks, hypertension, and fatigue among males. Poor diet, eating on-the-go, overwork, lack of exercise, and those ever-present family responsibilities are just a few of the stressors present in the lives of many men today. Others include use of tobacco, alcohol, steroids, antibiotics, and other chemicals. These elements contribute to nutrient depletion, which in turn puts more stress upon the body and decreases its coping ability. This vicious cycle can be broken with good nutrition, which can help to overcome destructive habits and addictions, and offset the harmful effects of other stressors.

## LONGEVITY AND MARRIAGE

Odds are six to one that a husband will die before his wife, though married men will likely fare better. Single men and widowers suffer more heart attacks, and their suicide rate is triple that of married men. Also, their life spans are shorter.

Perhaps the primary health benefit that men reap from the marriage relationship has to do with the nurturing they receive. The female of the species traditionally assumes this nurturing role, which literally involves providing nourishment for her family. It is her job to know about food, its selection and preparation.

And, of course, in the '90s the link between diet and health is well established. Women also provide emotional nurturing. They tend to worry about their men. While the single man may ignore a health problem and put off medical consultation, his married counterpart will likely seek medical advice sooner at the prompting of his worried spouse.

## MISGUIDED NUTRITIONAL MESSAGES

In April of 1992 the USDA adopted the Food Pyramid as a replacement for the traditional Four Food Groups. The guide recommends that carbohydrates—particularly breads, cereals, rice, and pastas—become the main focus of meals. Proteins like meat, fish, beans, and eggs are more of an accompaniment, not the main foundation. The category of fats, oils, and sweets is on top of the pyramid, indicating that we've got to go real light on these foods. You will see how you can suffer from this misguided information because certain kinds of fats are absolutely essential, not tangential, to the prostate, heart, and weight control. Unfortunately, this lopsided view of healthy eating has perpetuated the high-carbo eating that can be correlated with America's growing pot belly.

## HEADED IN THE RIGHT DIRECTION

Whether motivated by loss of health or the desire to prevent illness, enhance performance, improve appearance, increase longevity, please his woman, or some combination of these or other factors, men are actively seeking to improve their health through nutrition. Not only is nutrition a potent weapon for preventing disease and extending lifespan, it is also an excellent tool for achieving overall wellness as you will discover in *Super Nutrition for Men*.

The truly healthy male is one who is able to sustain a high level of energy, while cultivating calmness and focus at the same time. He is emotionally stable, mentally lucid, and physically fit. He is well nourished.

The real challenge in our Information Age then becomes wading through tons of nutrition books (all with diametrically opposed philosophies on how to achieve good nutrition), sorting this all out, and then finding a simple way to make practical use of the newly found information. Needless to say, this can be difficult, time-consuming, and confusing.

## TAKE UP THE CHALLENGE

Applying the no-hassle health and nutrition guidelines given in this book may take away the confusion, but will still require motivation and commitment. I remember reading the words of a physician, writing about men's health issues, who stated that he is typically harder on men than on women: And, he says, it works, for approached honestly, men will take up a challenge. Consider *Super Nutrition for Men* as an open invitation to take up the challenge and take charge of the lifestyle modifications that will change and maybe even save your life.

# CHAPTER 2

# LEAN & MEAN:
# CUT THE CARBS; ADD THE FAT

Cut the carbs, add the fat? Yes! I'll introduce you to the details of a dietary formula that does just that. It works for most men most of the time and can be modified to meet individual needs. This formula is a special mix of fats, carbs, and protein, designed to switch the body into a fat-burning mode. It calls for 40 percent of total calories to be derived from carbohydrates (like bread, pasta, and potatoes), 30 percent from natural and unprocessed fats (such as butter and olive oil), and 30 percent from protein (like low fat cottage cheese, turkey, water-packed tuna, eggs, fish, chicken, lean beef). Many men can expect to improve lean muscle mass on this program in as little as thirty days, trimming body fat to the ideal 14-18 percent range.

The program was pioneered by Barry Sears, Ph.D., formerly of the Boston School of Medicine and M.I.T. Sears's 40/30/30 approach has been successfully used by world-class athletes for over five years. Independent studies from Pepperdine University and Sansum Medical Research Foundation in Santa Barbara, CA, have demonstrated that the 40/30/30 formula not only improves athletic performance significantly, but also raises the level of the "good" cholesterol (HDL), is safe for diabetics, and aids in weight loss.

Cut the carbs; add the fat. Over the last decade, "expert" advice has directed us to do just the opposite—and during that time, the average weight of Americans has increased by ten pounds. Nonetheless, the "eat more/weigh less" mantra continues to echo through our homes, offices, and gyms. It has led to excessively high-carbohydrate diets, with sometimes as much as 70 percent of calories coming from carbohydrates. We appear to be growing fat on the low-fat, high-carbohydrate diet, with the average man carrying around 21-28 percent body fat. I'll show you why such a diet, while it might work for some men, will likely lead the majority not only into a condition of overweight, but also one of blood sugar instability that can sap vital energy and dull the mind.

No one diet will work for all men all of the time simply because everyone is biochemically unique. That uniqueness is shaped by ancestry, genetic heritage, and metabolic rate, all of which must be taken into consideration in personalizing a diet plan.

Whether a weekend warrior, professional athlete, sports enthusiast, or couch potato, every man wants to be strong and solid. Most believe that the best way to achieve an ideal body is through exercise. While exercise certainly has numerous benefits (see Chapter 10) and can indeed be a valuable adjunct tool in body shaping, it may surprise you to learn that diet is just as important, for two reasons:

1. Food consumption triggers release of the hormones that determine whether we will **store** excess body fat or **burn** it.
2. Due to their hormonal effect, food choices can reduce or enhance the benefits of exercise.

While overconsumption of carbohydrates, due to their sugar component, may have the **immediate** effect of increasing energy by raising blood sugar, the long-term result will be the lowering of sugar levels, with the resulting fatigue that is characteristic of hypoglycemia (low blood sugar). The ultimate consequence can be development of a more severe blood sugar disorder, like diabetes. In fact, the incidence of Type II (adult onset) diabetes has increased alarmingly in recent years, especially among blacks and Hispanics. Over six million American men now suffer from diabetes, while an estimated three million have early signs of the disease. So, America has been growing sick and tired—and fat—as a result of the low-fat, high-carbohydrate craze.

## THE HORMONAL EFFECT OF FOOD

Loosing weight on the high-carbohydrate diet can be difficult for some men, keeping it off even harder. And, worst of all, the bulk of weight

loss comes not from fatty tissue, but from muscle. Endocrinology studies over the last thirty years have shown that the proportions of
macronutrients—fat, protein, and carbohydrate—will determine
whether we store fat or burn it. With the right mix of macronutrients,
you can become a fat-burning machine.

The unsuspected key to successful fat-burning is the hormone insulin.
And insulin levels are controlled by the amount of carbohydrates in
the diet. When we consume carbohydrates, the pancreas secretes
insulin, which makes it possible for glucose (blood sugar made from
the sugar in carbohydrates) to enter the cells and be converted into
energy. Insulin prevents blood sugar from rising too high after a meal.
It is a storage hormone: It is responsible for the storage of excess blood
sugar in the liver (as glycogen) and in the muscles. Glycogen storage
capacity is limited. Once it is exhausted, the body will **convert excess
carbohydrate to fat** and store it under the direction of insulin.

Insulin is one of two hormones that is critically important in blood
sugar control. The other is glucagon, released when protein is consumed. Glucagon's action is the opposite of that of insulin. They are
inversely paired hormones—when one is high, the other is low.
Glucagon is a mobilization hormone. When the blood sugar level
drops (and with it, energy level), glucagon is secreted by the pancreas,
causing glycogen (stored sugar) to be released from the liver to replenish the sugar supply in the blood. Glucagon release also raises energy
levels by increasing the **release of fat from fat cells.** So, insulin lowers
blood sugar and stores fat, while glucagon raises blood sugar and mobilizes fat from storage.

| INSULIN | GLUCAGON |
|---|---|
| lowers blood sugar | raises blood sugar |
| stores fat | mobilizes fat from storage |
| triggered by carbohydrates | triggered by proteins |

Obviously, too much insulin will sap energy and increase body fat.

## MACRONUTRIENT BALANCE

So, as I've said, while carbohydrate consumption raises insulin levels
and lowers glucagon, protein consumption does the opposite: It raises
glucagon and lowers insulin. This is where the need for macronutrient

balance comes in to balance hormones. Fats enter the picture in that they affect the production of a group of little-known hormones called eicosanoids. Though their importance has been recognized only recently, eicosanoids are the oldest known hormones and, like glucagon, they are fat-burning friends when the right kind are released. They are said to act only upon the cell that produces them or upon an adjacent cell and are known to exist for only a few **seconds.**

Therefore, unlike the better-known hormones, eicosanoids cannot be measured. They encompass natural body chemicals with such exotic names as leukotrienes, thromboxanes, and prostaglandins. These substances regulate every cell in the body and are essential to every life form on the planet. These vital, but elusive, hormones are made from the essential fatty acid (EFA), linoleic acid. It is not just EFA intake however, but **everything** else that is eaten as well, that will determine the amounts and ratios of the **different kinds** of eicosanoids generated from the linoleic acid. Simply stated, there are "good" (series-1) and "bad" (series-2) eicosanoids. Their functions may be summarized as follows:

| "GOOD" Series-1 Eicosanoids | "BAD" Series-2 Eicosanoids |
|---|---|
| Dilates blood vessels | Constricts blood vessels |
| Anti-clotting | Clot forming |
| Bronchial dilatation | Bronchial constriction |
| Control cell proliferation | Increase cell proliferation |
| Strengthen immunity | Weaken immunity |
| Anti-inflammatory | Pro-inflammatory |
| Reduce cholesterol synthesis | Increase cholesterol synthesis |
| Anti-depressive | Increase triglyceride synthesis |
| Decrease pain | Increase pain |
| Stimulate endocrine hormones | |

Good eicosanoids regulate the cardiovascular system and control the mobilization of stored body fat. Our diet—the balance of macronutrients in it—will determine the ratio of good to bad eicosanoids. An excess of series-2 eicosanoids can lead to:

| | |
|---|---|
| fluid retention | pulmonary embolism |
| high blood pressure | asthma |
| heart attack | allergies |
| stroke | cancer |

thrombophlebitis                    infections
atherosclerosis                     connective tissue disease
autoimmune disease

In fact, "every known symptom and disease process requires an excess
of series-2 (eicosanoids)."[1] The most important dietary factor in determining a favorable eicosanoid balance is protein/carbohydrate ratio.
Overproduction of series-2 eicosanoids directs from excessive carbohydrate intake and inadequate intake of dietary protein. According to
research, the ideal ratios are reflected in the 40/30/30 formula. A significant alteration of these percentages at any meal can throw off hormonal balance. And, if carbohydrate levels are too high, body fat will
be stored and blood sugar lowered.

Jay Robb, a California-based fitness consultant and author of *The Fat
Burning Diet* (Loving Health Publications, 1994), knows first-hand
about the problems associated with a low-fat, high-carbohydrate diet
and the advantages to be gained from cutting the carbs and adding the
fat. Robb spent sixteen years searching for the perfect diet to control
his hypoglycemia. After numerous bouts of trial and error, he hit upon
a diet plan that not only controls blood sugar, but also assists in fat-
burning. He now advocates a diet that, is low in natural carbohydrates,
and contains adequate protein and healthy fat. He promotes this diet
through his "fat-burning seminars." According to Robb:

> The body is designed to use carbohydrates as fuel only
> temporarily. When we return to natural fat burning—
> which is what you're doing before you have that cere-
> al and fruit for breakfast—all insulin is controlled.[2]


## CARBOHYDRATE LOADING

With today's emphasis on "carbohydrate loading" for athletes, a
typical diet often consists of 70 percent carbohydrate, 15 percent
protein, and 15 percent fat. This kind of fuel mix elevates insulin
levels and therefore encourages hypoglycemia with attendant lack
of concentration. Fat is stored and any of the health problems associated with unfavorable eicosanoid production can develop. Such
effects would obviously impair athletic performance and provide
the biochemical scenario for the cyclist who "bonks," the marathon

runner who hits the wall, or the tennis player who loses his focus after a few hours.

The more desirable 40/30/30 balance of macronutrients allows the body to access its primary source of muscle energy, fatty acids, which are stored in adipose tissue (body fat). On a high-carbohydrate diet, this stored fat is not easily accessed, and the muscles must instead use carbohydrates, an inferior fuel, as a source of energy. According to Dr. Philip Maffetone, applied kinesiologist and trainer/coach for professional athletes (including top triathletes Mark Allen and Mike Pigg), fat provides over twice the energy of carbohydrates. Athletes are missing the boat with their high-carbohydrate intake: "The average U.S. athlete has a career span of four and a half years. . . .This is what happens when you rely on your sugar reserves, not fat reserves."[3]

When Maffetone first began working with Mark Allen, the Ironman Champion was running a seven-minute mile. Eleven years later he was doing 5:10-minute miles and doing them at a lower heart rate. During this period of time, the athlete actually became physiologically younger, according to Maffetone. Becoming both faster and younger are results that Allen credits to the way he trains, which includes following the 40/30/30 eating plan.

The higher proportion of energy obtained from fat with the 40/30/30 balance of macronutrients results in the conservation of muscle glycogen that, in turn, keeps blood sugar levels elevated, thus improving concentration and focus and endurance of athletes. Beneficial effects of the 40/30/30 diet include:

> increased lean body mass
> enhanced cardiovascular endurance
> increased burning of fat
> improvement of memory
> reduction of fatigue
> decreased hunger
> increased mental alertness

Many of the beneficial effects are attributed to the release of growth hormone from the pituitary gland that is stimulated by good (series-1) eicosanoids. Growth hormone builds and repairs muscle tissue.

Exercise can help us shape up and lose weight by cutting back insulin levels in the blood; however, loading up on carbs just before or after exercise will nullify the benefit due to the insulin response it evokes. More on this in Chapter 10.

## BALANCED MEALS

To obtain the full benefits of the 40/30/30 formula, you will need to follow it at **every** meal and at snack time as well. This is not a difficult task once the "how to" of applying the concept is grasped. Toward this end you will find meal planning guidelines in Chapter 11. These guidelines give sample meals, as well as tips to help you make your own balanced food selections.

Since the benefits of this approach to macronutrient balance were determined through studies with athletes, the area of sports nutrition has been the first to make practical application of the principles. One company, Bio-Foods, has sponsored studies showing the efficacy of this approach to eating and they have developed a tasty nutrition bar appropriately named "Balance."* Comprised of this 40/30/30 ratio of macronutrients, it is a definite contrast to most sports and energy bars that usually contain 75-90 percent carbohydrates. Balance bars can be used as a meal replacement, though they should not substitute for more than one meal a day. They also provide good appetite control—three to five hours for most people—on only 180 calories.

The stabilization of blood sugar that results from proper macronutrient balance helps control hunger and allows one to function optimally on less food (and therefore fewer calories) than normally consumed. The advantages for weight control are obvious. There is also the potential benefit of increased longevity; animal studies have repeatedly correlated reduced food intake with increased life span. When macronutrient consumption is balanced, reduced food intake does not correlate with hunger: Satiety is more readily acheived naturally.

## THE INSULIN RESPONSE

Hormonal balance is a key to health maintenance and/or restoration. Since food elicits hormonal responses that can be beneficial or detrimental, it is advisable to cultivate the habit of conscious eating. We

---

* The Balance nutrition bar is available through Bio-Foods 1-800-678-4246.

need to be aware of the effect our food choices will have—not only upon our health—but upon our appearance and mental state as well. Bear in mind the hormonal responses that are triggered by the intake of carbohydrates and proteins:

| **Insulin Release Triggered By Carbohydrates** | **Glucagon Release Triggered By Proteins** |
|---|---|
| lowers blood sugar | raises blood sugar |
| produces "bad" eicosanoids | produces "good" eicosanoids |
| stores glucose as glycogen, remainder as fat | mobilizes fat |

Carbohydrate overloading tends to displace protein foods needed by the body for immunity, stable blood sugar level, hormones, and tissue repair. Additionally, carbohydrates such as bread, pasta, and potatoes are deficient in EFAs needed for the production of good eicosanoids. The overconsumption of carbohydrates, with its subsequent stimulation of the insulin response, can lead to:

| | |
|---|---|
| weight gain | food cravings |
| bloating | cardiovascular disease |
| fatigue | |

Carbohydrates include a wide variety of foods that are rich in sugars or complexes of sugars. All plants—fruits, vegetables and grains—fall into the carbohydrate category. Carbohydrate overload most often takes the form of excessive consumption of grains, especially wheat. Evidence exists that prior to the agricultural revolution, some 10,000 years ago, our ancestors subsisted on more protein and less carbohydrates than we do today—i.e., a diet approximating the 40/30/30 macronutrient ratio. They did not eat grains or dairy products.

Changes in our diet have outpaced genetic adaptations. Our digestive systems have not evolved sufficiently to accommodate the incorporation of large amounts of grain. Wheat represents over 80 percent of our total grain consumption. Gluten, a plant protein found in wheat, rye, oats, and barley is not handled well by an increasing number of individuals. Though heredity plays a role in "gluten intolerance" (also known as sprue or celiac disease), diet is the initiating factor.

In gluten-sensitive individuals, the plant protein damages the lining of the intestines, causing malabsorption. The body's inability to fully utilize vitamins and minerals leads to development of the any of the following symptoms: diarrhea, anemia, muscle spasms and cramps, bone or joint pain, headache, bloating, and intestinal pain. Gluten-intolerant men can substitute such grains as rice, millet, and buck-wheat.

Another problem with grains—especially wheat, rye, and oats—is their high phytic-acid content. Phytic acid, a phosphorus-like compound, interferes with calcium absorption and limits absorption of iron, magnesium, and zinc as well. It is concentrated in grain husks. So, even healthy whole grains can provide high levels due to their bran content. Commercial breads also contain phytic acid in their yeast.

Overconsumption of carbohydrates, paired with underconsumption of essential fats, contributes to the proliferation of the yeast germ, Candida Albicans, and to the development of hypothyroidism and adrenal insufficiency. These are all common conditions today that can lead to food allergies and sugar cravings. These conditions, in turn, aggravate the problem further by depressing the body's ability to metabolize carbohydrates.

## NOT ALL CARBS ARE CREATED EQUAL

The arrangement of sugars in carbohydrates determines whether the food is "simple" or "complex." Simple carbohydrates are readily digested and found in sugars and fruits. Complex carbohydrates, on the other hand, have a more elaborate molecular structure, being made up of rows of sugars. They are found in vegetables, as well as whole grains, beans, and legumes. The high-fiber content of these foods helps slow the release of sugar into the bloodstream. The reasoning has been that because they take longer to digest, they don't play havoc with blood sugar and insulin levels, as simple sugars can do. Therefore, complex carbohydrates have been frequently recommended for control of hypo-glycemia.

What is not well recognized, however, is that some complex carbohydrates have a very high glycemic index, which means that they convert quickly to blood sugar and therefore raise insulin levels rapidly. The Glycemic Index compares how rapidly carbohydrates are converted to blood sugar compared to glucose which is given an index of 100 percent. Surprisingly, certain complex carbohydrates have a higher glycemic index than some simple sugars as indicated in the following examples:

| RAPID | MODERATE | SLOW |
|---|---|---|
| rice cake  133 | spaghetti  60 | apples  39 |
| whole wheat bread  100 | pinto beans  60 | yogurt  36 |
| brown rice  82 | sucrose  59 | lentils  29 |
| banana  82 | oatmeal  49 | peaches  29 |

Because of their higher glycemic index, rice cakes eaten alone will increase insulin levels much more rapidly than peaches. (Refer to Chapter 11 for a more complete glycemic index.) Any of the complex carbohydrate made from grains (even whole grains) such as rice cakes, pasta, bread, bagels, and puffed cold cereals will react more like a simple sugar in the body because of the processing that the original gain has undergone. Eating the whole grains themselves (in the form of buckwheat, barley, millet, etc.) will, on the other hand, cause a slower release of glucose into the bloodstream.

Generally speaking, we want to choose foods with a low glycemic rating, (especially if they are to be eaten alone) to achieve sustained energy and appetite control. The overall glycemic response of the carbohydrates eaten at a meal will be influenced by the other foods consumed at that meal. Proteins and fats will both slow down insulin release. While the consumption of rice will increase insulin levels significantly, the chicken you eat with it and the olive oil on the accompanying salad will reduce the overall glycemic response of the rice and that of any other carbohydrates present in the meal.

The glycemic rating of a food is based upon its digestibility, quality of its fiber, and amount of time that it is cooked. Cooking raises a food's glycemic index since it makes starch more digestible. Instant rice cooked for one minute has a 65 percent rating, cooked for six minutes, a 121 percent rating.

In consideration of this information, we would do well to favor complex carbohydrates from legumes and vegetables, such as lentils, garbanzo beans, corn, and squash in our diet and avoid overloading the system with grains. We will also want to select protein-rich nuts and seeds as snacks, rather than insulin-stimulating crackers, breads, and muffins.

## FAT PHOBIA

It was fat phobia that gave birth to the carbohydrate craze of the last decade which has, by no means, been limited to athletes. Fat phobic individuals are everywhere. They're often motivated by desire to lose weight and decrease the risk of developing heart disease, still the number one killer in this country. Many avoid such basic nutritional staples as meat, eggs, and butter due to erroneous information they've received about cholesterol and fat. Instead, they fill up on sugar which, ironically, **will** cause them to gain added pounds **and** increase their risk of developing cardiovascular disease (see Chapter 6).

Fats serve vital functions in the body. They are required for hormone production. They facilitate oxygen transport; lubricate and insulate muscles and organs; aid in the absorption of fat-soluble vitamins (A, D, E, & K); nourish the skin, mucous membranes, and nerves; and help maintain body temperature. Without fat in our bodies, we would die instantly. Our cell membranes and nervous system would collapse.

It is, of course, possible to overdo the fat consumption, and many Americans do. As nutritionist, Robert Crayhon, puts it: "Too much fat is a problem, but so is too much brown rice, exercise, or water. Anything in excess is unhealthy."[4] The fact of the matter is too little fat can cause problems too. Animal studies have shown that deficiencies in essential fatty acids can result in eczema and sterility. A deficiency of these essential fats can also cause inflammation; dry, flaky skin; acne; and arthritis, as well as other symptoms. Overweight, too, is linked with EFA deficiency, for in the absence of essential fatty acids, the body converts sugar to fat much more rapidly. This causes blood sugar to drop and appetite to escalate, giving rise to overeating.

Also, EFAs move "bad" fats out of the body. They emulsify and move saturated fats and cholesterol through the bloodstream and out of artery and tissue deposits. Regardless of the quantity of fat consumed, if the **quality** is poor, health problems will develop. Poor quality fat consists of fat lacking in essential fatty acids, which includes fats and oils that have been refined. The Standard American Diet (SAD) of overprocessed fast foods, excessive sugar and salt, and insufficient fiber and essential fats abounds with such poor quality fats.

While a diet composed of 30 percent poor quality fats will most certainly cause problems, one composed of 30 percent good fats—unrefined monosaturates (such as olive and canola oils), and unrefined polyunsaturates (natural vegetable oils and certain fish oils)—can be very beneficial.

Most of these fats provide EFAs that control the cardiovascular, repro-ductive, and nervous systems and are crucial to the functioning of the immune system. Without EFAs, cell membranes weaken, making the body vulnerable to infection. The essential fats also retard the entry of carbohydrate into the system, thus keeping insulin levels lower.

Essential fatty acids, once referred to as vitamin F, are those that the body cannot make. They must be supplied in the diet. They include two groups of polyunsaturated fatty acids—the Omega-3s and Omega-6s—that serve vital body functions. In addition to serving as precursors to eicosanoids, EFAs also regulate cell membrane fluidity and function and are believed to have enzyme-like functions or to be co-factors in enzymes.

Recent research has found that over 20 percent of adults, as well as many children and infants have EFA abnormalities. Studies have shown that people on a highly fat-restricted diet can show extremely low levels of Omega-3s—less than 5 percent of normal in some cases. Illness also creates a dramatically increased need for these EFAs. The following is a list of conditions known to correlate with Omega-3 defi-ciencies. It was compiled by Dr. Bruce West and appeared in the March 1995 edition of his *Health Alert* newsletter:

| | |
|---|---|
| AIDS | obesity |
| alcoholism | pregnancy/breastfeeding |
| B-vitamin deficiencies | renal transplants |
| neurological disease | retinitis pigmentosa |
| cirrhosis | Reye's syndrome |
| coronary occlusion | rheumatoid arthritis |
| coronary artery disease | scleroderma |
| Crohn's disease | sepsis (infection) |
| head injury | Sjogren-Larsen syndrome |
| kidney disease | skin disease |
| lupus | vitamin E deficiency |
| multiple sclerosis | Wiscott-Aldrich syndrome |

## THE OMEGAS

The original Omega-6 fatty acid is linoleic acid. From it, our bodies produce gamma-linolenic acid (GLA). Alpha-linolenic acid is the origi-nal Omega-3 fatty acid. From it our bodies make eicosapentaenoic acid (EPA) and docosahexaenoic acid (DHA):

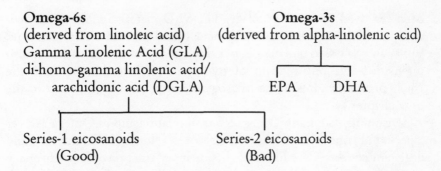

**Omega-6s**
(derived from linoleic acid)
Gamma Linolenic Acid (GLA)
di-homo-gamma linolenic acid/
    arachidonic acid (DGLA)

**Omega-3s**
(derived from alpha-linolenic acid)

EPA        DHA

Series-1 eicosanoids
(Good)

Series-2 eicosanoids
(Bad)

You'll note that the series-1 and -2 eicosanoids derive directly from DGLA and arachidonic acid respectively, both of which are derivatives of GLA. Arachidonic acid comes from red meat; therefore, eating too much of it can produce bad eicosanoids.

Basically, your Omega-6s and -3s are found in the following foods:

| OMEGA-6 LINOLEIC ACID | OMEGA-3 LINOLEIC ACID |
|---|---|
| vegetable oils | cold-water fish (like salmon, mackerel, |
| legumes | sardines, tuna, herring, anchovies) |
| all nuts and seeds | wild game |
| and most grains | flax seed and flax oil |
| breast milk | canola oil |
| organ meats | walnuts |
| lean meats | pumpkin seeds, chia seeds |
| leafy greens | soybeans |
| borage | wheat sprouts |
| evening primrose oil | fresh sea vegetables |
| gooseberry and | leafy greens |
| black currant oils | |

You'll recall that the eicosanoids are made from linoleic acid and that prostaglandins fall into the eicosanoid category. Prostaglandin research is ongoing. They are involved in such vital processes as blood clotting, inflammation, hormone production, pain perception, and smooth muscle contraction. As members of the eicosanoid family, there are "good" and "bad" prostaglandins. The balance of Omega-6 to Omega-3 oils is critical to proper prostaglandin metabolism.

This balance is upset in the Standard American Diet (SAD), which is composed largely of processed foods from which Omega-3s have been removed to retard spoilage. The SAD diet also tends to be deficient in EPA, an Omega-3 fatty acid found in cold-water fish, wild game, and flax seed and canola oils. Deficiency of this fatty acid is also intensified by consumption of hydrogenated fats that produce the "bad" prosta-glandins. (The hydrogenation process is discussed in the next chapter.)

Consuming too many Omega-6 fats in relationship to Omega-3s over a period of time will increase the risk of developing inflammatory and degenerative disorders like arthritis, urinary tract disorders, coronary artery disease, lupus, or multiple sclerosis. We can correct this imbalance by adding more Omega-3s from the food sources listed above. An overabundance of Omega-3s can be a problem too: It can cause excessive bleeding, while Omega-3 deficiency can lead to excessive clotting and artery obstruction. The higher the ratio of Omega-3 to Omega-6, the less likely that a clot will obstruct the artery.

Flax seed oil is the best vegetable source of the Omega-3s. Its consumption helps to oxygenate the body. It can be used liberally in salad dressing and/or substituted for butter over vegetables and grains. It cannot, however, be used for cooking, as it is very heat sensitive. Canola oil, a monounsaturated oil, is another good vegetable source of Omega-3 fatty acids. It was developed in Canada from the rapeseed plant. Canola has a mild taste and may be used on salads, for baking, and for low-heat recipes. I've mentioned that Omega-3s and -6s are "polyunsaturated" fatty acids. Let me now clarify exactly what that means.

## CLASSIFICATION OF FATS

"Saturated," "polyunsaturated," and "monounsaturated" are chemical terms which refer to the way in which hydrogen is carried in the fatty acid molecule. They relate to the type and number of hydrogen bonds in the chemical structure of the fatty acid. All fats contain a combination of these three types, with one predominating. Basically, saturated fats carry more hydrogen than unsaturated ones. The three different types of fats have distinct characteristics and are predominate in different foods as indicated on the next few pages:

## SATURATED FATTY ACIDS (SFAS)
**Have straight molecules.**
**Are solid at room temperature.**
all meat fats
dairy products
coconut oil
cocoa butter
palm oil
palm-kernal oil

## MONOUNSATURATED FATTY ACIDS (MUFAs)
**Have one kink or bend in their molecules.**
**Are liquid at room temperature, but solid when refrigerated.**
olive oil
almond oil
apricot kernel oil
peanut oil
canola (rapeseed oil)
high-oleic safflower oil
high-oleic sunflower oil

## POLYUNSATURATED FATTY ACIDS (PUFAs)
**Have two or more kinks.**
**Are liquid even when refrigerated.**
These fats are the Omega-3s and -6s listed on page 19.

While canola oil is chiefly a monounsaturated fat, it is also a source of Omega-3s, as previously mentioned. The Omega-3s actually lower triglycerides and the level of "bad" cholesterol (LDL) in the body. Adults need a total intake of two to five tablespoons of EFA-rich oil daily. Most of this amount can be obtained from food—whole foods, not refined ones. Generally I recommend supplemental amounts of EFAs—one tablespoon of flax seed oil per day for the Omega-3 it provides and one tablespoon of unrefined safflower oil or 4 capsules of GLA from evening primrose oil as a source of Omega-6.

While saturated fats, found primarily in animal products, have gotten the reputation of being "bad" fats because of their connection with high cholesterol and hardening of the arteries, they are, in fact, of themselves not bad at all. Moderate amounts of saturated fats, when consumed **in balance with** the essential fatty acids and a full spectrum of other nutrients and in the absence of artificial fats, are not problematic in the healthy body. (See Chapter 6 for a discussion of the cholesterol issue.) Too much saturated fat in the bloodstream, however, can prevent the blood from supplying sufficient EFAs to the organs that need them, creating a relative EFA insufficiency.

Replacing saturated fat with essential fats will lead to a healthier, leaner body. EFAs are burned up in the body faster than other dietary fats and their presence is vital in the diet if weight loss is to be achieved. One EFA in particular, GLA activates the fat-burning process.

Jeff, a forty-two-year old overweight male who believed he was doing everything right could not lose a pound. He had read *Beyond Pritikin* and called my office to inquire whether he, a male could go on the same program as his wife. She was following a lower carbo diet and adding GLA in the form of Evening Primrose Oil to her regimen. She not only lost her desired seven pounds, but also several inches around her waist. I encouraged Jeff to follow a similar program and get on the GLA pronto. Three weeks later Jeff wired a dozen roses to the office with a note: "Thanks—One rose for every pound lost."

## THE QUESTION OF BALANCE

It's plain to see from the foregoing that without sufficient essential fatty acids of both the Omega-3 and -6 varieties, it will not be possible to achieve balance in the diet. It is conditions of imbalance on both a chemical and energetic level that create fatigue, weight problems, and disease. Achieving hormonal balance through proper eating allows us to regain our health and achieve our genetic weight. The 40/30/30 eating plan is designed to re-establish this balance and no doubt will work wonders for many people, perhaps the majority. Let us bear in mind, however, that studies demonstrating its efficacy were carried out primarily on athletes and we may not be able to generalize the results to the public-at-large. In truth, I believe that there really is no **one** diet that is best for all people.

While I've been pretty hard on the low-fat, high-carbohydrate diet as a panacea for every man, I must admit that for some, it may be therapeutic, at least in the short run. However, I do believe that for others, its net results will be counterproductive for the reasons enumerated in previous pages. Just as a diet too heavy on carbohydrates can be deleterious to the health, so can one too high in proteins or too high in fats. Balance is the key. However, what puts one man in balance might throw another off, given our "biochemical individuality."

The Pritikin diet, very high in complex carbohydrates and low in fat and protein has had its success stories. So too has the Atkins diet, very low in complex carbohydrates, but high in protein. These radically different diets both have had beneficial results—**but not with the same people.** What are the factors then which determine what type of diet is best suited to our highly individual nutritional needs? There are three major ones which I'll discuss briefly here. For more detailed information, refer to my book, *Your Body Knows Best* (Pocket Books, 1996).

## ANCESTRY

Though the diet of humankind has undergone radical changes over the last forty thousand years, genetically, we have changed very little in that time. It has been the climate of the land that has been the prime determinant of the foods available in it. Our ancestors, over time, naturally adapted to changes in their environment and the diet it dictated. Those adaptations were genetically encoded in our lineage and therefore ethnic and genetic conditions persist regardless of how much people move around. Studies have demonstrated that the best diet for an individual is that of his or her native culture. Someone of American Indian heritage does best on a Native American diet of beans, squash, cactus, or buffalo, even if he moves to Japan. Changing location does not change our genetic/nutritional needs.

Basically, we can think of our ancestral heritage in very broad terms, as indigenous to either northern or southern climates. The north encompasses Scandinavia, Canada, and northern and eastern Europe. These cultures adapted to diets high in cold-water fish, red meat, and root vegetables. The diet of southern locales featured light meat, fish, tropical fruit, beans, legumes, and light, water-based vegetables, such as lettuce, tomatoes, peppers, and cucumbers.

Because of the "melting pot" nature of our culture, most Americans have a mixed genetic heritage. Therefore, the genetic blueprint of our nutritional needs may not be that easy to decipher. For this reason, ancestry becomes a secondary consideration in determining optimal diet, with the primary factor being metabolic type.

## METABOLIC TYPE

Your metabolic type is based upon you oxidation rate—the rate at which you turn fuel (food) into energy. In the '70s, a psychologist, Dr. George Watson identified two types of oxidizers: fast and slow. I refer to them as fast and slow **burners.** What these two categories of people have in common is that neither uses energy efficiently.

The slow burner doesn't process food quickly enough (**under**active adrenals and thyroid), whereas it is speedily converted to energy in the fast burner (who has **over**active adrenal and thyroid glands). The slow burner gravitates toward simple carbohydrates, sodas, and sugary foods for energy and tends to binge on starches. Generally, the appetite is poor and there is a dislike for protein-rich foods and fats.

The fast burner, on the other hand, will feel hyper, anxious, and irritable without sufficient fat and protein in the diet. The appetite is generally strong, with a preference for heavy meats. The emotional state is often characterized by peaks and valleys—as energy levels fluctuate. While the slow burner tends toward poor circulation, low blood pressure, and dry skin, the fast burner is usually warm, perspires easily, and has high to high-normal blood pressure.

The slow burner does best on a diet emphasizing protein and, to a lesser extent, carbohydrates (which, of course, should not be overconsumed). Protein can increase metabolism 30 percent, while a pure carbohydrate meal increases it only 10 percent. Animal proteins of the lean variety (cod, tuna, eggs, and poultry) should be consumed at two meals each day. Purine-rich proteins, such as organ meats, are to be avoided and fat intake should be modest, as it will further slow down the metabolism.

The fast burner does best on a diet emphasizing fats and protein. The heavier meats should be favored, with beef, lamb, venison, or cold-water fish eaten with every meal. These foods add substance and help balance out the highs and lows of the fast burner. Fats help slow down the overactive metabolism. Purine foods can be eaten freely. Both fast and slow burners should avoid processed carbohydrates such as bread, pasta, bagels, muffins, and crackers.

Not all people fall into these two categories. Some are normal or mid-range burners. They are generally able to maintain a desirable weight, due to their metabolic efficiency, whereas weight gain can be a problem for both the fast and slow burner. Eating in such a way as to restore metabolic balance helps to normalize weight and eliminate disease conditions.

Metabolic type can be established through hair analysis. Questionnaires can also help a person determine his oxidation rate, as can increased awareness of the body and its response to food. The questionnaires below will assist you in establishing your metabolic type and help in formulating a more personalized dietary plan. Answer "yes" or "no" to each question:

## SLOW-BURNER QUESTIONNAIRE

1. Are you somewhat laid back and even-tempered? _____
2. Does red meat feel heavy in your system? _____
3. Do you approach problems one step at a time, rather than juggling many things at once? _____
4. Can you skip breakfast without losing energy or getting hungry? _____
5. Do sweet things like candy or fruit give you a quick pick-up? _____
6. Do you prefer a "light" meal of salad and pasta rather than a "heavier" one of steak and potatoes? _____
7. Do you get thirsty a lot? _____
8. Do foods like cheese, butter, and avocados seem to make you feel sluggish? _____
9. Does coffee start your morning off just right? _____
10. Do you feel you need a pick-up from spices and particularly enjoy tangy condiments like mustard, ketchup, and salsa with your food? _____

## FAST-BURNER QUESTIONNAIRE

1. Do you consider yourself high strung or feel hyperactive? _____
2. Do you actually feel better eating a plate of chops rather than leaner eats like chicken? _____
3. Do you enjoy a hearty high-protein breakfast (eggs and bacon)? _____
4. Do you reach for salty snacks like nuts or potato chips when you are stressed out? _____
5. Are avocado, cheesy sauces, and full-fat dairy products very satisfying to you? _____

6. Do you feel better eating full meals every two to three hours?

_____

7. When you eat sweet foods like cakes and cookies, do you burn out quickly after a short energy burst? _____
8. Do you have a hearty appetite? _____
9. Does drinking coffee make you nervous? _____
10. Does a pat of butter on toast satisfy you more than jam? _____

If you answered "yes" to 8 or more questions in the slow-burner questionnaire, you are a classic slow burner type.

If you answered "yes" to 8 or more questions in the fast-burner questionnaire, you are a classic fast burner type.

Fast burners will do best on the 40/30/30 eating plan, while slow burners may feel better if they increase carbohydrates just a bit and lower the fats. If you fall in-between these two types, your current diet is probably serving you well.

## BLOOD TYPE

The different blood types are related to the movement of generations of people over the continents. They appeared at different times in our evolutionary cycle, type O being the oldest type on the planet. Type A appeared next, then B, followed by AB. The oldest types (O and A) are the most common in our culture today, with 85 percent of Americans falling into one or the other of these two categories. The most rare type was the last to evolve, type AB, which encompasses only 4 percent of our culture. Nutritional needs evolved along with blood types as follows:

TYPE O—　　Adapted to a diet heavy in animal meat and fish. Doesn't do well with dairy or excessive grains. Tends to have an active lifestyle.

TYPE A—　　Best suited to semi-vegetarian diet (lean meat, poultry several times a week) due to a genetic lack of HCL. Doesn't handle dairy well. Shouldn't overdo grains. Less active than type O.

TYPE B—　　Can handle a wide variety of foods (both A and O diets). Can do dairy in moderation—fermented milk probably best.

TYPE AB—    The only type fully adapted to dairy products. May
            have some type-A characteristics with less tolerance
            for meat and animal products.

From the above, we can see that certain blood types would have a difficult time on a diet low in animal protein, while others would do
much better on it. While most people in our culture have adapted to
eating meat to some degree, few are able to handle dairy from the
point-of-view of blood type. It should be added that there are two sub-
types of A, one better adapted to meat-eating than the other.

The information on blood type and diet is fascinating. Research is
ongoing, particularly in Japan, home of the world's foremost authority
on the subject, Toshitaka Nomi.

## WHERE TO START?

Start with your metabolic type. Once you know whether you are a fast
or slow burner, then you can modify your diet based upon blood type
and ancestral heritage. If any of these factors are unknown, work with
the information you have. Use the 40/30/30 eating plan as a point of
departure, regardless of other factors, modifying the diet as would be
appropriate in terms of what is known about ancestry, metabolic type,
and blood type.

The appeal of the 40/30/30 plan is that it avoids extremes of too
much or too little in terms of percentages of macronutrients. Diets that
*are* extreme can at times be a blessing to the person for whom they're
appropriate. But extreme diets should only be temporary diets. In the
long run, they may move the person past the point of balance into
imbalance. And for those who are already out of balance, an extreme
diet will push them further out of balance and can be very damaging.

The Standard American Diet is approximately a 51/37/12 formula—
51 percent refined carbohydrates, 37 percent saturated and bad fats, and
only 12 percent protein. The protein content is inadequate in relation
to the overabundance of fat and carbohydrates. For good health you
need to bring this into balance and switch to quality foods.

## WHAT ABOUT LEAN MUSCLE MASS?

While men seem to handle a larger carbohydrate load than women (probably due to greater muscle mass and fewer fat cells), the basic hormonal response to food is not gender specific. Men are no less vulnerable to the problems resulting from carbohydrate overload. Some men, however, **will** lose weight on a grain or pasta-based regime—**lots of weight.** They often lose more weight than they need to (and with it, muscle mass), and they're constantly hungry because they don't metabolize the grain protein well and don't absorb enough nutrients from the food. They often overeat, prompted by constant hunger, but the more they eat grains, beans, and vegetables, the thinner they get.

Such a diet, devoid of meat, eggs, and dairy, will often lead you into a serious shortage of protein and essential minerals. You will sense that you are missing something, and feel a lack (which really is a state of diminished nutrition) that creates a desire for sweets. When you give in to these cravings, you will **then** begin to put on fat. This same cycle can be brought on by diets that include some meat, but are deficient in good oils.

Over the years, nutrition authorities and writers like Robert Atkins, M.D., John Yudkin, M.D., William Dufty, and Cass Ingram, M.D., have warned that sugar and starches (carbohydrates) can sabotage weight loss and set the stage for degenerative disease. The high-carbohydrate craze has born witness to the wisdom of their warnings. See Chapter 6 for more information on sugar.

Following a balanced eating plan—appropriate to your biochemical individuality—will assist you in ridding the body of unwanted fat. I use the word "fat" instead of "weight" because the two do not necessarily correlate: Muscle weighs two and a half times what fat weighs. One can lose inches and look trimmer while maintaining the same weight or even putting on pounds.

It is highly recommended that you have body fat measured before beginning the balanced eating plan and then again in thirty to sixty days. This can be done in several ways: By measuring skin-fold thickness on various parts of the body with calipers, through hydrostatic (or underwater) weighing, or through bioelectrical impedance which measures the body's resistance to a low-frequency alternating current.

How much fat will be lost depends upon four variables:

1. The amount and type of carbohydrate consumed
2. The present level of fitness
3. The amount of calories expended
4. The amount of calories taken in

As previously indicated, total calorie intake should decrease with the 40/30/30 eating plan as appetite decreases.

Arnold, a thirty-four-year-old fitness buff, came to see me complaining that he could not lose weight even though he was working out daily and following what he believed was a healthy diet. Arnold believed in carbohydrates. After doing an extensive dietary assessment it was obvious that he also believed in the "more is better" theory. Arnold's diet consisted of enormous amounts of carbohydrates—like dry cereal, bagels, pasta, potatoes, fat-free muffins, and pita bread— eaten morning, noon, and night and in-between. After explaining to him the value of the 40/30/30 formula for weight loss and peak performance Arnold agreed to include lean protein like eggs, white fish, and skinless turkey at every meal. He also agreed to add some butter to his bread and flax oil to his baked potatoes. He agreed to stop his gargantuan portions of carbos. He also learned to choose his carbos from the lower end of the glycemic index. Within three weeks, Arnold was burning fat and losing inches.

George, a forty-two-year-old office manager was also having difficulty losing weight when he came to see me. He too had been following the high-carbohydrate/low-fat diet, but was not prone to exercise. After initially losing some weight on this diet, he had begun to gain it back. He told me he felt lethargic and craved sugar constantly. He felt totally out of control when it came to his eating. His dietary assessment revealed a shortage of good protein and a total lack of good fats. George thought he was doing the wise thing by cutting back on meat and eggs and consuming margarine and the "no cholesterol" vegetable oils from his local grocery store. But his body was starving for protein and healthy fats that level blood sugar and help control sugar cravings. Once we added back butter and olive oil to his diet, upped his protein intake, and cut back on the carbs, George began to lose weight again. And now that he has more energy he started working out in the gym.

On the low-fat/high-carbohydrate diet, very little of the weight lost is fat, for the insulin response bars access to the body's fat depots. Eating a diet of balanced nutrient composition, adequate in protein, on the other hand, spares glycogen stored in muscles and the liver, and burns fat, rather than storing it. Protein triggers the release of glucagon and drives the metabolism. With inadequate amounts, the body is hampered in its fat-burning ability.

Men need a higher ratio of protein than is contained in the Standard American Diet. This increased protein need is due to a metabolism that is tilted toward tissue breakdown (catabolic). During sex, men discharge large amounts of stored protein, carbohydrates, and minerals. Men also tend to lose weight with greater ease, due to operating at a higher metabolic rate to maintain a larger percentage of muscle mass. Read more on protein in Chapter 4.

The challenge for today's man is not one of losing weight through dieting, but rather one of getting healthy. This can be accomplished while building muscle and shedding fat through exercise coupled with the application of the principles of nutrition outlined in this chapter. Following such principles equates more with adopting a healthy lifestyle than "going on a diet": a bigger challenge perhaps, but one with more rewarding and long-lasting benefits.

## THE BOTTOM LINE

Major points to remember from this chapter include:

You can build lean muscle mass, shed fat, increase energy, endurance, and mental performance by following the 40/30/30 eating plan at every meal.

You can activate your body's fat-burning mechanism by increasing the amount of protein and good fats in your diet, while reducing carbohydrate intake.

Your food choices will control the levels of beneficial hormones produced in your body—and thereby impact your health and well-being.

Your metabolic rate, genetic heritage, and blood type provide clues to your individual dietary needs.

# CHAPTER 3

# QUALITY COUNTS

## REFINING

The refining of grain was made possible by the invention in 1862 of machinery that removes and disposes of the outer husks of the grains. It is in these outer husks that most of the nutrients are concentrated. Typically, in the production of flour, the bran and germ are removed, resulting in extensive losses of nutrients.

During the First World War, the milling of grains was forbidden in Denmark due to economic cutbacks. The death rate fell 34 percent and the incidence of cancer, kidney disease, and diabetes dropped significantly. During the Second World War when grains were only partially milled in England, much the same thing happened. The less we refine food, the more it supports our health.

Among the nutrients lost in the refining process are the B vitamins, a family or "complex" of vitamins that plays an important role in nourishing the nervous system. We need extra amounts of the entire B family when we're under stress, but refined products, even though "enriched" with a few of the Bs put back, can't meet this need. A continuous diet of refined food cripples the body's ability to deal with stress, a prominent feature in the life of today's man.

Also lost in the refining process are many of the important "antioxidant" nutrients—vitamins A, C, and E and the minerals selenium and zinc—so necessary for their role as "free-radical" scavengers in the body. Free radicals are renegade chemical fragments caused by such

31

stresses as pollution, oxidation, exposure to ultraviolet radiation, ingestion of rancid oils, and surgery. They are believed to play a key role in
aging and in the degenerative disease processes, particularly cancer.
Men need antioxidant nutrients to protect their bodies against damage
from free radicals. Consuming a diet of refined foods creates deficiencies in these important protective nutrients and therefore increases vul-
nerability to degenerative diseases.

Also lost in the refining process is fiber, needed to move food residue
through the intestines and prevent constipation. Many of the vitally
important trace minerals are lost, as well. According to Henry A.
Schroeder, M.D., who did extensive research on the trace minerals over
twenty years ago, "most of the energy in the average American diet
which comes from white flour, white sugar and fat, is not supplied
with the trace substances needed to utilize that energy efficiently and
properly."[1] The refining of sugar removes 93 percent of the ash and
with it, the trace minerals needed to metabolize the sugar. The milling
of wheat into refined white flour and the refining of raw cane sugar
into white sugar remove minerals in the following percentages, according to Dr. Schroeder:

|            | white sugar | white flour |
|------------|-------------|-------------|
| chromium   | 93 percent  | 40 percent  |
| manganese  | 89 percent  | 86 percent  |
| cobalt     | 98 percent  | 89 percent  |
| copper     | 68 percent  | 83 percent  |
| zinc       | 98 percent  | 78 percent  |
| magnesium  | 98 percent  | 85 percent  |

Additionally, white flour has lost the following minerals originally present in whole wheat: 60 percent of the calcium, 71 percent of the phosphorus, 77 percent of the potassium, 78 percent of the sodium, 76 per-
cent of the iron, 48 percent of the molybdenum, and 75 percent of the
selenium.

Iron is the only mineral that is later added back to food when it is
"enriched." It is put back in an inorganic form, iron sulphate. Inorganic
iron taken into the body stays out of solution. The body is unable to
absorb it properly. The absorption problem is compounded by the
lack of other minerals in refined foods. As a consequence, this iron
often ends up being deposited in the arteries and joints, leading to
degenerative disorders like heart disease and arthritis. Enriching foods

with iron can cause more problems than it solves. In Sweden liver cancer rates tripled when they began fortifying their flour with iron.

While inorganic forms of iron are not well absorbed, natural iron supplements, such as iron peptonate, are—especially when electrolytes are balanced. The "heme" form of iron found in animal products is also well utilized, making liquid liver extract a good supplemental source of iron for those who need it.

Iron deficiencies among men are rare, however, except possibly among those who have low thyroid function, have lost blood, have been ill, or have engaged in endurance exercise. If in doubt about iron levels, have laboratory tests performed, but as a general rule men should avoid taking supplemental iron and consuming foods enriched with it, for iron overload can create serious problems including heart disease, arthritis, diabetes, and impotence. Also, excess iron is stored in the central nervous system and is found in many psychiatric patients. High levels of the free form of the mineral are found in the brains of those suffering with Parkinson's Disease. See Chapter 6 for more on information on iron, iron overload, and how to detect it.

Following the refining process which removes most of the eight vitamins present in whole wheat, only three are replaced in the "enriching" process. All together, refining removes over two dozen nutrients and replaces only four.

White "polished" rice is also a refined product. After processing, it retains only the following percentages of trace minerals present in the whole grain: 17 percent of the magnesium, 25 percent of the chromium, 73 percent of the manganese, 62 percent of the cobalt, 75 percent of the copper, and 25 percent of the zinc. Choose brown rice over white for a more nutritious meal.

When we remove bran and germ from whole wheat, nothing is left but the starch. It is in the starchy portion of the grain that the heavy metal, cadmium, is concentrated. Cadmium toxicity is strongly associated with hypertension. If enough zinc is present in the body, it can defend against the cadmium. Unfortunately zinc is found in the bran and germ portions of the grain, and is discarded in processing. This means that when we eat refined grains, we are vulnerable to the ill-effects of cadmium, particularly if our body stores of zinc are low. This is not a problem with the whole grains. In the absence of chromium and fiber, also removed in the refining process, the body has trouble processing the starch that remains. Pure starch stresses the pancreas and throws the blood sugar into turmoil.

Most of the oils consumed in the Standard American Diet are highly refined. According to Schroeder, separating oil from corn results in a refined product with less than 1 percent of the magnesium and only 25 percent of the original zinc. Vitamin E, needed to help retard spoilage, is also removed, as is lecithin, a fat emulsifier. The fat-digesting enzyme, lipase, is destroyed by the heat used in processing, making the oil undigestible. Beta carotene is also virtually destroyed by processing methods. And, perhaps worst of all, refining destroys much of the valuable Omega-3 and Omega-6 EFAs.

## MANLY MINERALS

Many of the most important minerals for men are largely discarded in the refining process. Some, like selenium are all but absent from our soils. The minerals most needed by men include:

**Zinc:** This mineral is the most crucial in that it is intricately tied up with male potency, fertility, and sex drive. The more sexually active the man, the more he needs zinc. Ejaculation spends 420 micrograms of the stuff. Other kinds of physical activity have the same result, since minute particles of zinc pass through sweat. Low zinc levels have been linked to low semen volume and to low levels of testosterone. Zinc supplements can be helpful in treating benign prostate hypertrophy (BPH) that commonly afflicts men over fifty. Found primarily in red meats, eggs, and seafood, beneficial amounts range from 15-50 milligrams per day. Zinc picolinate seems to be best utilized.

**Calcium:** Men who consume lots of calcium tend to have lower blood pressure and less hypertension. Calcium is necessary for building bones. One-third of all hip fractures occur in men. Rich calcium sources include dairy, leafy greens, sea vegetables, and fish bones. The recommended dose is from 800-1,500 milligrams per day. Calcium citrate is well absorbed.

**Copper:** Copper is a double-edged sword. On the one hand, copper is a warrior in defense against heart disease and problems with steady heart rhythms. Copper deficiency can raise cholesterol and blood pressure and lead to problems maintaining heart rhythms. On the other hand, copper excess is a common problem these days due to dental fillings, water pipes, and adrenal depletion. Copper toxicity can be an underlying cause of panic attacks and yeast infections. It is found in soy products, regular tea, cocoa, nuts, peas, beans, and oysters. About two milligrams a day is the recommended amount.

**Chromium:** An estimated three million men are walking around with early signs of diabetes without knowing it. Chromium can protect against full-blown diabetes by boosting the body's ability to regulate blood sugar levels. It is also a noted fat-burner and can help in attaining lean muscle mass. Two tablets of brewer's yeast will supply a day's need of chromium. Amounts from 200-800 micrograms are beneficial.

**Magnesium:** Those men headed for the gym will need to keep their stores of magnesium intact. This mineral plays a critical role in muscle activity. It also helps protect against heart disease, which kills more than 350,000 men each year. It is great for high blood pressure and acts like a natural tranquilizer. It is found in green leafy vegetables and nuts like almonds and seeds. Recommended amounts range from 600-1,000 milligrams per day.

**Selenium:** This is a disease fighter credited in the fight against cancers of the skin, lung and stomach that kill more than 100,000 men yearly. It pairs with vitamin E to protect cells from damage by oxygen-containing free radicals. Per day amounts range from 100-400 micrograms.

## FOOD PROCESSING

Americans today get 70 percent of their calories from non-nutritious foods, including:

    35-40 percent from damaged fats
    20 percent from refined sugars
    10 percent from alcohol

Fats become damaged when they're overheated or hydrogenated. Hydrogenated oils and refined sugar are foods that have undergone commercial processing. Food-processing procedures include refining, enriching, preserving, and irradiating. This is done to our foods for the sole purpose of extending their shelf life. None of these processes enhances the food nutritionally. To the contrary: They result in considerable loss of nutrients.

Among the most heavily processed of our foods today are oil and grain products—these include all kinds of salad oils, cooking oils, and shortenings, breads, pastas, and pastries—anything made with white sugar and/or white flour. One of the most fundamentally important changes a single man can make in his shopping and eating habits is to buy only unrefined oil and grain products. Look for these in your local health food store or in the "special foods" section of your supermarket. Select oils labeled "unrefined" or "expeller pressed" and breads made with "whole wheat flour." Many labels simply say "wheat flour," which is a deceptive name for white flour, which is, of course, made from wheat.

## ENRICHING

We have already touched on the enriching process which puts back a small portion of the vitamins and minerals refined out of foods and noted that those minerals put back are in an inorganic form which is not well utilized by the body.

Iron is replaced in the enriching process, but copper, needed for its utilization, is not. Unabsorbed iron adds to the body's storehouses and can be especially problematic for men. Ultimately, all nutrients work synergistically and when one or more is removed from the whole food, the activity of those remaining is adversely affected. Enriched food, in a sense, is like N-P-K fertilizer: Both provide only a small portion of the full spectrum of nutrients needed for optimal health, growth, and strength.

Nutrient deficiency predisposes both plant and human to disease conditions. Crops become infested with insects and then are treated with chemical pesticides. We medicate our sick soils in much the same way as we medicate ourselves when our bodies are invaded with germs, **our** form of "bugs." In both instances, the "bug" problem may well be averted by providing the host with nutrient-dense food—for the plant that is natural fertilizer, such as rock dust, and for humans, it is food grown on soils fertilized in this manner, "organic" foods.

## GO ORGANIC

Organically grown foods, those grown without the use of chemicals, show minimal toxicity and provide superior nutrition. They are becoming increasingly popular. In 1994, there were 3,000 more certified organic farmers in this country than there were in 1990.

There is great variation in the mineral content of vegetables grown in different locations and under different conditions. Variable soil quality makes for variable food quality. The Firman Bear report, originally issued through Rutgers University in 1948, shows just how great these variations can be.

**THE FIRMAN BEAR REPORT**
*Rutgers University*
**VARIATIONS IN MINERAL CONTENT OF VEGETABLES**

| | Calcium | Magnesium | Potassium | Sodium | Manganese | Iron | Copper |
|---|---|---|---|---|---|---|---|
| **SNAP BEANS** | | | | | | | |
| Highest | 40.5 | 60 | 99.7 | 8.6 | 60 | 227 | 69 |
| Lowest | 15.5 | 14.8 | 29.1 | 0 | 2 | 10 | 3 |
| **CABBAGE** | | | | | | | |
| Highest | 60 | 43.6 | 148.3 | 20.4 | 13 | 94 | 48 |
| Lowest | 17.5 | 15.6 | 53.7 | 0.8 | 2 | 20 | 0.4 |
| **LETTUCE** | | | | | | | |
| Highest | 71 | 49.3 | 176.5 | 12.2 | 169 | 516 | 60 |
| Lowest | 6 | 13.1 | 53.7 | 0 | 1 | 9 | 3 |
| **TOMATOES** | | | | | | | |
| Highest | 23 | 59.2 | 148.3 | 6.5 | 68 | 1938 | 53 |
| Lowest | 4.5 | 4.5 | 58.8 | 0 | 1 | 1 | 0 |
| **SPINACH** | | | | | | | |
| Highest | 96 | 203.9 | 257.0 | 69.5 | 117 | 1584 | 32 |
| Lowest | 47.5 | 46.9 | 84.6 | 0.8 | 1 | 19 | 0.5 |

Millequivalents per hundred grams / Trace elements ppm

Since this report is almost fifty years old and mineral depletion of the soils has greatly increased in the intervening years, we can assume that today's figures would be even lower than those cited above. Study this chart. It should give great impetus to "go organic."

## PRESERVING

The FDA has approved some 2800 food additives. These include chemicals added to our foods to flavor, color, stabilize, thicken, and emulsify them. Preservatives retard spoilage by checking the growth of micro-organisms. One has to wonder if these foods cannot support the health of micro-organisms, how can they possibly support the health of larger organisms like us?

Among the preservatives widely used in our foods to retard spoilage are sulfites, benzoates, nitrates, and nitrites. Benzoates are the most commonly used of the preservatives. Sulfites are found in beer, wine, and dried fruit. Both of these preservatives can cause allergic reactions and should be avoided by those who are allergy-prone.

Sodium nitrate and nitrite are used widely today in curing meat and smoking fish. Packaged meats containing sodium nitrite should be avoided, for in the stomach, nitrites combine with amines (products of protein break down), forming nitrosamines, known carcinogens. The nitrogen from chemical fertilizers is another source of nitrates. Seepage into underground aquafers can contaminate drinking water supplies. Vegetables, too, can absorb too much of the fertilizer and pass nitrogen compounds on to humans. Bacteria in the stomach convert these to deadly nitrites. When nitrites enter the bloodstream, they react with hemoglobin to form methemoglobin. The resulting disease, methemoglobinemia, causes the victim to turn blue from lack of oxygen. Suffocation and death may result, especially in babies.

Benjamin Feingold, M.D., found that a large percentage of hyperactive children are unusually sensitive to preservatives and to artificial colors and flavors. He found a link between food additives and learning and behavioral disorders. Hyperactivity is today becoming better known as ADD, Attention Deficit Disorder. ADD affects a number of adults, as well as children, and is commonly treated with counseling, behavioral modification techniques, and drugs. Since drugs destroy nutrients, deepening deficiency, they can aggravate the problem by increasing sensitivity to adverse effects of food additives. Dietary restriction of food additives is certainly a safer and most likely a more effective approach, as demonstrated by the success of the Feingold diet. Choose whole foods whenever possible to avoid preservatives and other food additives.

## HYDROGENATION

You'll recall that the terms saturated and unsaturated refer to the degree of saturation with hydrogen and that saturated fats, coming from animal fat and tropical oils, carry more hydrogen. Despite their bad reputation, saturated fats, consumed in moderation and in balance with other dietary components, will do no harm in the healthy body. The harm comes from the altered, damaged fats Americans routinely consume. Over the last century, the rise in cardiovascular disease (350 percent) has paralleled the rise in both sugar and processed oil consumption and has not correlated with cholesterol consumption which has remained about the same.

For years, the myth abounded (and still persists) that substituting margarine for butter is the "heart smart" thing to do. The reasoning has been that, because margarine is made from unsaturated vegetable oil, it is better for us than butter, an animal fat that is more saturated (with hydrogen). What is not realized is that margarine is created from unsaturated oils that are hydrogenated.

Hydrogenation was first developed in 1912 by a Frenchman who created it as a means of hardening soap. The process involves supersaturating oil with hydrogen at temperatures exceeding 400 degrees F., using nickel as a catalyst. Hydrogenated corn, soy bean, safflower, or canola oil are a much greater health risk than are naturally saturated fats such as butter. The harm caused by these oils is not only in their hydrogenation which destroys nutrients, including those needed for a healthy heart—vitamins E and $B_6$ and the minerals chromium and magnesium, but also in the Trans Fatty Acids (TFAs) that are formed as a result of it.

The TFA molecule is strictly man-made, does not appear in nature, and consequently the body has difficulty metabolizing it. Because vegetable oils start out with a low level of hydrogen, it takes a long time to saturate them through hydrogenation. During this time, the harmful trans fats are formed. Tropical oils, on the other hand (palm, palm kernel, coconut, and cottonseed), start out with a high level of hydrogen saturation and so it takes much less time for them to become hydrogenated and TFAs do not form in the process. These fats, therefore, need not be eliminated from the diet if they are regulated by the inclusion of essential fatty acids. It has been found, in fact, that countries with high intake of tropical oils have a significantly lower risk of cardiovascular disease, hypertension, and cancer than the U.S.

A special word should be said here about cottonseed oil. Because cotton is a "non-food" plant, numerous herbicides, pesticides, and fungicides are sprayed on the plants. Residues of these poisons can be found in the seed and in the oil from the seed. I recommend that cottonseed oil be avoided in the diet. Once again it is important to read the labels, because partially hydrogenated cottonseed oil is one of the major ingredients of processed and packaged foods.

TFAs tend to stay in the blood where they increase serum cholesterol. A study printed in the British medical journal, *The Lancet* (March 3, 1993), suggests that a high intake of trans fats may increase the risk of coronary death by 50-67 percent.

TFAs tend to increase LDL (the so-called bad cholesterol) and decrease HDL (the good). No one knows for certain what level (if any) of TFAs can be safely tolerated by the body, but many researchers feel that amounts in excess of two grams per day should be avoided. Here's a list of TFA levels found in common foods:

| Food | TFAs in grams |
|------|---------------|
| cookies, chocolate chip, snack pack | 11.54 |
| Imitation cheese—American sliced | 8.07 |
| Milano cookies (small bag) | 6.65 |
| 1 large Danish pastry | 6.63 |
| 1 sugared donut | 5.28 |
| 1 apple turnover | 5.23 |
| crackers, 10 small, (partially hydrogenated soybean oil) | 4.36 |
| margarine, 1 tbs. | 3.5 |
| vegetable shortening, 1 tbs. | 2.7 |
| butter, 1 tbs. | 0.5* |

Notice that the two-gram limit is easily exceeded in the SAD. Consuming as little as three to four grams per day of TFAs can lead to a 30 percent increase of cardiovascular disease. Industry officials and the Federal government claim that Americans take in eight to ten grams of TFAs daily. Fat expert Dr. Mary Enig of Silver Springs, M.D., thinks this is an underestimate. She believes we eat between 11 and 28 grams per day, which would be about 20 percent of total daily fat intake.

To avoid TFAs, it is necessary to eliminate vegetable shortenings, margarine, processed cheeses, commercial baked goods, mayonnaise, candy bars, processed peanut butters, and microwave popcorn from the diet. Make a habit of reading labels and avoiding anything that says "hydrogenated" or "partially hydrogenated."

*Information taken from *Trans Fatty Acids in the Food Supply: A Comprehensive Report Covering 60 Years of Research* (Enig Associates, Inc., 1993) by Mary G. Enig, Ph.D.

Apart from the damage done directly by TFAs, these altered fats also block the pathways used by the essential fatty acids, leaving the body deficient even when these good fats are part of our diets. This can adversely affect cell function and depress the immune system.

The evidence clearly shows that the real "heart smart" thing for you men to do is to avoid hydrogenated vegetable oil products like the plague and get into the EFAs big time.

## ELECTROLYTES

Electrolytes are mineral salts that can conduct electricity when dissolved in solution. In the body, the bloodstream provides the fluid medium for electrolyte formation. It is the electrical energy conducted by electrolytes that runs the body. Electrolyte deficiency or imbalance results in energy loss, leaving us feeling fatigued—a common complaint. And no wonder, considering the scarcity of the vital trace minerals, necessary for electrolyte formation in the body.

Fatigue is the first symptom of just about everything. When we have insufficient energy to run the body, its processes break down. Electrolyte balance then is crucial to our health. Without it, we cannot maintain homeostasis. Homeostasis is the body's balancing mechanism. Again that word "balance," so vital to our health. When it is disrupted at any level, energy flow is disturbed and chemical processes adversely affected, leading to development of disease conditions. Henry A. Schroeder, M.D., tells us in *The Trace Elements and Man* (Devin-Adair, 1973) that homeostatic mechanisms will break down under two conditions:

1. deficiency of vital trace elements
2. excess of vital elements

Deficiencies, as I've discussed are widespread today, owing to the depletion of our soils (and food processing, discussed earlier), so we won't find our food supply to be a reliable source of trace minerals.

## WHAT ABOUT WATER?

Two of the most effective ways to purify our water is to use distillation or reverse-osmosis methods, both of which remove minerals, as

well as pollutants. If you use these methods, then you're going to
need to add trace minerals back to the water. However, most liquid
mineral formulas on the market are colloidal in nature. Colloidal
minerals are inorganic. They are not capable of osmosis (cannot fully
penetrate cell walls) and therefore are not well utilized by the body.
Additionally, many come from sources that are contaminated with
heavy metals.

Cultures that enjoy exceptional health and longevity drink mineral
water that cascades down from mountain streams and swirls over
rocks, creating vortexes. This whirling motion generates an electrical
charge in the minerals taken up by the water, changing them from a
colloidal to a much more bioavailable crystalloid form. In this manner,
nature creates electrolytes, which are fully assimilated by the body,
owing to their crystalloid form.

We can duplicate nature's electrolyte formation by adding crystalloid
minerals back to our purified water. A liquid mineral supplement containing the correct minerals in the correct amounts and in a crystalloid
form constitutes a true electrolyte formula. The only such formula
available on the market today, to the best of my knowledge, is a product called Trace-Lyte.* Regular use of this product will help restore
electrolyte balance.

Restoration of electrolyte balance will assist the body in combatting
virtually any disorder by eliminating conditions which gave rise to it.
Among those basic conditions is pH imbalance which can be corrected
through the regular use of Trace-Lyte, in combination with a balanced
diet. Diet alone cannot regulate pH, however, in the face of electrolyte
imbalance. PH balance is one of the body's major defenses against disease. Another is osmotic equilibrium, the equalization of force or pressure between the inside and outside of cell walls. The restoration of
osmotic equilibrium strengthens cells and makes them unfit hosts for
bacteria and other germs. This restoration is accomplished by re-estab-
lishing homeostasis through electrolyte balance.

## ELECTROLYTE BALANCE

Electrolytes must be in balance for certain beneficial bacteria to exist
and carry out their function of fighting harmful bacteria. The proper
functioning of the immune system depends upon electrolyte balance.

*Trace-Lyte is available through Uni-Key 1-800-888-4353.

Many scientific papers written in the last twenty years indicate that by restoring pH and osmotic equilibrium, we may lower significantly the risk of infection. In addition to normalizing pH and osmotic pressure, electrolytes also help to restore peristaltic action of the bowel muscles, increase digestive efficiency, increase oxygen to the cells, reduce water retention problems, correct neuro-muscular imbalances, improve enzyme production, regulate blood sugar levels, increase energy levels, and strengthen the immune system.

While inorganic forms of minerals may form deposits in various organs and tissues of the body, causing such problems as kidney and gall stones, "hardening" of the arteries, constipation, and arthritis, the crystalloid form will not do so. In fact, it will actually help eliminate existing deposits by creating balanced conditions that allow the minerals to go back into solution. Crystalloid minerals, as electrolytes, likewise play an active role in "escorting" heavy metals out of the body. They are nature's own chelators.

Trace-Lyte can be used as an electrolyte supplement, and it can also be used to re-mineralize purified or distilled water; add one teaspoon to each gallon.

Taken in conjunction with other nutritional supplements, it will enhance their activity by improving assimilation. If very large amounts of isolated minerals are taken over a long period of time, however, we run the risk of disrupting balance once again, since excessive mineral intake as well as deficiency can cause a breakdown of homeostatic mechanisms.

Overabundance of some minerals can create deficiencies of others. Ideally, we want to incorporate mineral-rich whole foods, such as sea vegetables, into our diet, as a highly usable and balanced source of organic minerals. Sea vegetables include nori, dulse, hijiki, wakame, arame, kombu, and agar-agar and are good in vegetable soups and natural jellos.


## QUALITY COUNTS

As I said before, "quality counts." In order to choose quality macronutrients for peak performance it is necessary to be able to discern just what constitutes good quality in the world of food. Quality foods include fruits and vegetables grown organically, meat obtained from organically raised animals, "fertile" eggs laid by chickens that roam free, sea vegetables, whole grains, and unrefined oils. Quality beverages include fresh fruit and vegetable juices, herbal teas, and purified water to which electrolytes have been added.

Packaged, canned, and bottled items should be avoided as much as possible and never be purchased without first checking the label, even in a health food store. Avoid artificially sweetened foods and all products containing hydrogenated or partially hydrogenated oils, as well as commercially processed dairy products, packaged meats, and smoked fish. Shop the outside aisles of your supermarket—where the whole foods are—and patronize your local health food store.

## MARS BARS, MINUTE RICE, AND MARGARINE: A FLAWED STUDY

In doing the research for this book, I ran across a scientific study that stopped me dead in my tracks. It focused on the effects of carbohydrates and fats on energy levels in the human body. What was appalling about it was that the carbohydrates fed to the subjects in the study consisted of minute rice and Mars bars and the fat used was margarine. All of these are highly processed foods, altered from their natural state. The resulting nutrient loss makes them fragmented foods that react very differently in the body than do natural, whole foods. Processed foods are unbalanced in their nutrient composition and therefore create imbalances in the body, disrupting normal physiological processes and leading to disease conditions. To draw conclusions about how the body responds to carbohydrates and fats in general based on how it responds to these unnatural, devitalized ones in particular is not accurate and can give rise to the formulation of erroneous data.

The potential benefits of the 40/30/30 formula cannot be realized if you eat a diet made up of 40 percent refined carbohydrates, 30 percent hydrogenated fats, and 30 percent protein from animals who do drugs. The benefits of the big three macronutrients, carbohydrates, fat, and protein are seriously compromised when micronutrient (vitamin and mineral) content is altered, as it is in today's foods. That's why quality counts.

## IN CONCLUSION

Important facts to remember include the following:

We can compensate for nutrient loss from soil depletion and food processing by choosing organically grown whole foods and using food supplements.

Regular use of a true electrolyte formula can help restore homeostasis or balance to the body. This will assist in the prevention of disease conditions and aid in recovery from all types of illness.

# CHAPTER 4

# PROTEIN MAKES A COMEBACK

Lean protein: the white meat of poultry, flank steak, eggs, and fish, is a cornerstone of super nutrition. It can make the difference between optimum male nutrition and **mal**nutrition. Protein, which comes from a Greek word meaning first, is appropriately named because it is the most important of the macronutrients, found in virtually every cell of the body. Eating enough of the right kind of protein can transform your body into a fat-burning machine and give you extended energy, improved concentration, and appetite control.

I remember way back to the '70s when we were advised to eat as much protein as possible. Nutritionist Adelle Davis had us counting protein grams instead of calories. By the '80s, we were loading up on carbohydrates in preference to proteins, wary of cholesterol problems we were taught would result from eating high-protein meat and dairy products.

The pendulum has swung one way, then another. And now, it seems it has moved toward the middle, the point of balance. As we have come to recognize the hormonal effects of food, the merits of protein are being examined in a new light. However, rather than a "more is better" approach, we're seeing the importance of balancing protein intake with carbohydrate and fat. We are learning that by increasing protein intake **in relationship to carbohydrates**, we trigger a favorable hormonal response.

Protein, as we learned in Chapter 2, activates the fat-mobilization hormone, glucagon, which assists us in losing weight, building lean

47

muscle mass, stabilizing energy levels, controlling hunger, and so forth. By increasing the protein to carbohydrate ratio to balance macronutrients, the appetite is normalized. Consequently so is caloric intake, which diminishes as hormonal balance is established. This is not a high-protein diet, for the actual **number of grams** of protein that we take in daily in the 40/30/30 eating plan might remain the same as it was before—or even decrease. Many men can adjust the ratio simply by reducing the carbohydrates in their diet.

## FUNCTIONS OF PROTEIN

In addition to the stimulation of glucagon production, adequate protein intake is needed for the following body functions:

tissue growth and repair
formation of neurotransmitters in the brain
stimulation of metabolism
a strong immune system
healthy hair, skin, and nails
building of new cells
regulation of fluid balance
muscular strength and tone
energy production and endurance
normal digestion
blood clotting
formation of hormones

Protein controls the catabolic/anabolic cycle of the body. In the catabolic phase of this cycle, muscle tissue is broken down during strenuous physical activity, whereas it is built up in the anabolic phase. Increasing protein intake in the diet facilitates the formation of new muscle. Muscles contain more protein than any other structure of the body. Men need more of it—and more calories—because of greater muscle mass and because their metabolism leans toward the catabolic.

## AMOUNT NEEDED

You need about 50 to 75 grams of protein per day. Individual needs vary, based upon nutritional status, body size, and activity level, as well as genetic factors. Athletes, especially body-builders, need more protein than less active men. To stimulate muscle growth, weight lifters should take in approximately 1 to 1½ grams of complete protein per pound of lean body weight, while endurance athletes require ⅔ to ¾ gram of protein per pound of lean body weight.

The Recommended Daily Allowance for protein intake for men is set at 56 grams. It has been estimated, however, that the average man consumes more than twice this amount daily—and still his protein consumption represents only 12-18 percent of total daily calories. Therefore, for most men, the challenge is not so much one of adding more protein grams, as it is balancing protein intake with carbohydrates and fats—and, of course, upgrading the quality of all macronutrients. There are problems associated with both underconsumption and overconsumption of protein.

## DEFICIENCY SYMPTOMS

Deficiencies of this vital nutrient may lead to abnormalities of growth and tissue development. The protein-deficient man often has poor posture since he lacks the muscle tone and energy to stand perfectly erect. He may also have a diminished sex drive, constant food cravings, thinning hair, and brittle nails. The mental state is often characterized by irritability, depression, and confusion. A study of MIT students found that protein significantly improved their ability to do mental tasks, while carbohydrates curbed this ability by making them more relaxed. Proteins produce two chemicals in the brain that boost alertness: dopamine and norepinephrine.

Because it boosts metabolic rate, increased protein intake can be especially beneficial to the slow burner, giving him more energy and better endurance. Increasing metabolism can help burn off stored fat and improve utilization of energy from foods.

The protein-deficient man may also be bloated and overweight due to insufficient albumin, a blood protein, that makes urine collection possible. Without adequate protein, sufficient albumin can't form and water leaks out from the cells into the spaces between them where it can't be excreted by the kidneys.

Insufficient protein can result in poor resistance to infection, impaired wound healing, and delayed recovery from illness. Antibodies are the body's chemical bullets for the fight against such pathogens as viruses and bacteria. An antibody is, by definition, a blood protein of the globulin type. Without adequate dietary protein antibodies can't form and immunity is impaired. Phagocytes (killer cells), a form of white blood cell important to our immunity, are also made of protein. So, too, are enzymes. Protein deficiency thus creates an inability to produce adequate quantities of enzymes. This adversely affects digestion, which in turn hampers the body in its ability to utilize other nutrients.

Roger, a twenty-five-year-old graduate student had begun eating a vegetarian diet after reading a very popular diet book in the late '80s that touted food combining and vegetarianism. For several years he felt marvelous. He had more energy and more mental clarity. Then slowly but surely, his energy levels reached a plateau and began to slip. He also began to experience reoccurring colds and bouts of flu.

After reviewing his high-carb, low-protein diet history, I immediately added fish and chicken to his eating program on a daily basis. Roger also agreed to include at least four eggs a week in his diet. He found a pick up in his energy almost immediately. And his bouts with colds and flu have subsided to one cold or so a year.

Protein builds new cells to replace those that are constantly lost from day to day, such as skin and hair cells. Stresses, such as injury, surgery, hemorrhage, and prolonged illness cause loss of body protein. Supplemental protein may therefore be indicated at times of stress; however, excessive protein intake may cause fluid imbalance and other problems.

## EXCESS IS BAD, TOO

Seventy-two percent of the protein consumed by Americans comes from animal products. A high intake of animal protein has been linked to osteoporosis and kidney stones. The link found here is in the effect of excess protein on calcium metabolism. When protein intake is increased from 47 to 142 grams daily, the excretion of calcium in the urine doubles.[1] Alkaline minerals (primarily sodium and calcium) are needed to buffer the acid ash left from consumption of meat. Usable forms of these minerals are obtained primarily from fruits and vegetables which are sparse in the SAD. According to Senate Document #436, published in 1936, 99 percent of Americans are mineral deficient!

Overconsumption of acid-forming foods, such as meat, forces the body to rob its own storehouses—to take sodium from the muscles and calcium from the bones and teeth—to provide alkaline mineral to neutralize the acid caused by excess protein consumption.

Paul and Mike were twenty-something weight-lifters who wanted to get real "mean and lean." They began following an extremely high-protein diet, consuming eight-ounce steaks twice a day. They believed that combining this with their weight-lifting would stimulate fat burning and build muscle mass. In a little less than a month on this overdose of protein, both came to see me on the recommendation of a friend. Paul had suffered a stress fracture in his right wrist, and Mike was constantly complaining about his whole body feeling tight, his lower back constantly aching.

It appeared that both these guys were forcing their bodies to rob their bones for calcium and their muscles for sodium. I immediately switched them to the 40/30/30 plan and put them on Trace-Lyte Electrolytes. I also advised both of them to choose fat-free cottage cheese to help replenish calcium and sodium reserves. Within eight days both reported feeling better, with a leveling of mood swings, and relief of lower back pain.

A high intake of animal protein has also been linked to heart disease, high blood pressure, and kidney disease. While excessive intake of saturated fats contained in animal products can be a risk factor in the development of coronary-artery disease; lack of EFAs, overconsumption of sugar, and macronutrient imbalance are perhaps more important, though less recognized, factors. I'll tackle the cholesterol question in Chapter 6, but just a word on it here: Cattle of today store a different kind of fat in their muscles than did the animals of yesteryear. These animals were range-fed on grasslands, but today they're fed grains and injected with the growth hormone, stilbestrol. Whereas the grass-fed cattle accumulated a fatty acid called oleic acid in their muscles, today's beef cattle store a different kind of fat, called stearic acid, which contributes to the elevation of LDL (bad) cholesterol.

## THE BASICS

Next to water, protein is the most plentiful substance in the body. Proteins comprise 50 percent of our body's weight. They are made up of amino acids, twenty-three of them. All contain nitrogen which other foods lack. When we eat protein-rich foods, the body breaks the protein down into its component amino acids. Thousands of proteins are made from different combinations of amino acids. Some are used by the cells to build new tissue, others to construct antibodies, hormones, enzymes and blood cells.

Of the twenty-three amino acids, eight are considered "essential," meaning that they can't be produced by the body, but must be supplied in the diet. These include:

| | | |
|---|---|---|
| tryptophan | lysine | methionine |
| phenylalinine | leucine | valine |
| threonine | isoleucine | |

Also, arginine and histidine are two amino acids that are essential in the growth period of life and sometimes, due to acquired or genetic factors, in adult life as well.

A food is considered a "complete" protein if it contains all of the eight essential amino acids. Complete proteins include meat, fish, poultry, milk, and dairy products. Bee pollen and spirulina also qualify. Of the meats, liver and kidneys have the highest protein value in terms of their amino-acid profiles.

High-protein meal replacement formulas are frequently used for weight loss and supplemental protein. Those containing casein should be avoided. Casein is a difficult-to-digest milk protein to which many men are allergic. Commercially it's used to glue wood together because of its tenacious adhesive quality. The casein content of cow's milk is three hundred times higher than mother's milk and a by-product of its bacterial decomposition is mucous production: Yet another strike against milk—despite the fact that it is a complete protein. Meat is a better choice for complete protein—meat from free-range chickens, wild game, and antibiotic and hormone-free beef.*

Eggs are also an excellent source of complete protein for men. They are one of the few food sources of the sulfur-containing amino acid, l-cysteine, which is essential for healthy skin, hair, and nails. Their cholesterol content should not be a concern, for high dietary cholesterol

*A company called Lean and Free (1-800-383-BEEF) raises hormone and antibiotic-free cattle. Their beef can be ordered by mail and shipped throughout the country. Other companies that provide organic beef include: Country B3R Meats (Childress, TX) and Coleman Natural Beef (Denver, CO). Organically raised chicken and turkeys from Shelton Farms, Harmony Farms, Foster Farms, and Young's Farms are sold through health food stores and cooperative buying clubs.

does not translate into high cholesterol in the body. **And**, eggs have a high lecithin content. As a fat emulsifier, lecithin is a cholesterol-lowering agent. One can safely eat eggs every day, though powdered eggs should be avoided. The cholesterol in powdered eggs is oxidized and therefore toxic to blood vessels.

Since soybeans are a complete protein, the vegetarian would do well to make liberal use of tempeh and tofu (soybean products) in his diet. (He should make sure, however, to supplement zinc to offset high copper levels in all soy products.) Soy's health benefits give the meat-eater a reason to incorporate it into his diet as well. The entire soybean family of plant chemicals provide protection against cancer, and any of the foods made from soy significantly lowers blood cholesterol and reduces the risk of heart disease.

Other excellent plant protein sources include honeybee pollen and sesame seeds. Bee pollen contains all of the amino acids, the essentials and the nonessentials. Its therapeutic effects include regulation of metabolism and oxygenation of cells. Many athletes and Olympic stars use it. As a supplement, 1 to 2 teaspoons can be taken daily with food or beverage. It is best to start with a smaller amount, say $\frac{1}{2}$ teaspoon, and increase gradually.

Another fine vegetarian source of complete protein is the blue-green algae, spirulina. It, along with bee pollen, is considered by many to be one of the world's most perfect foods. Spirulina is a rich source of natural protein (60-71 percent) that is more digestible than most foods because of its lack of cellulose. It is also rich in vitamins, minerals, and EFAs.

## FOOD COMBINING

It has traditionally been taught that in order to properly synthesize protein, the body must be supplied with all essential amino acids simultaneously in the proper proportions. For example, plant foods do not contain sufficient amounts of all of the essential amino acids. They are, therefore, considered to be "incomplete" proteins. Grains lack lysine and threonine, while beans lack methionine. By combining grains with beans at the same meal, the amino acid profile is complete.

This practice, however, is not in vogue anymore. Current teaching dictates that complementary proteins can be eaten during the course of the day rather than at the same meal. I am personally in favor of the current teaching for another reason: Eating grains and beans together can create an overload of carbohydrate, leading to excessive insulin production and its fat-promoting properties in sensitive individuals.

## TWO EXTREMES

Since both excess and deficiency of protein can cause problems; the heavy meat-eater and the vegetarian alike can be in trouble. Problems of the latter stem from deficiency, while those of the former result from toxicity. Consuming excessive amounts of meat in the absence of fiber-rich carbohydrates will cause constipation and putrefaction of protein, with resulting toxicity.

The deficiencies that can occur in a vegetarian diet are numerous, especially if the diet is vegan (devoid of eggs and dairy, as well as flesh products). Plasma and urine tests conducted at Aatron Medical Services reveal that vegetarians are commonly deficient in the amino acids lysine, methionine, tryptophan, carnitine, and taurine. The first three of these are essential amino acids. Lacking these, the body can develop immune and liver dysfunction, weight problems, and sleep disorders.

Also common among vegetarians are $B_{12}$ deficiencies, for this vitamin is found only in animal products. Pernicious anemia is the classic sign of $B_{12}$ deficiency, but other symptoms can include dementia, depression, paleness, and numbness and tingling in the extremities. The vegan should consider supplementing his diet with 500 micrograms of $B_{12}$ regularly.

Less well known is the fact that vegetarians also commonly lack zinc. This mineral is critical for proper immune, reproductive, and blood sugar functioning and, as previously mentioned, is one of the minerals most needed by men, if not **the** most needed. The typical vegetarian diet is high in copper. This can give rise to such conditions as skin problems, yeast infections, lowered immunity, schizophrenia, depression, and lack of mental focus.

## WHEN VEGETARIANISM IS APPROPRIATE

In consideration of metabolic type, ancestry, and blood type, I believe it's fair to say that a vegetarian diet is not appropriate for the majority of men. A man with blood type O who is a slow burner of Northern European heritage cannot maintain health on a vegetarian or even a semi-vegetarian diet. He may, however, find, as other types have, that such a meatless diet is effective as a **short-term therapeutic regimen**, particularly if it incorporates plenty of fresh vegetable juices. Vegetables contain a number of unique substances with healing properties, including carotenes, flavonoids, and chlorophyll, as well as thousands of phytochemicals. But most importantly, they provide high levels of minerals (vegetable juices especially) needed by the body to form electrolytes and reestablish homeostasis.

Since all other nutrients (including protein) require minerals for their activity, saturating the body with them through juicing (and, ideally taking Trace-Lyte) in times of illness becomes a priority. Because juices provide no fiber, however, it is also necessary to eat whole vegetables themselves. The fiber helps to detoxify and build up the body. Once the body is built up to the point where digestion is normal (through restoration of pH balance provided by the electrolytes and the alkaline ash of the vegetables), extra protein is needed to build new tissue and complete the healing process. To provide high-protein foods **prematurely**, however, simply adds to the body's toxic burden. Without the digestive ability to break the protein down into its amino acid components, it will putrify and thus postpone recovery, rather than assist it.

If high-protein foods of animal origin are not added back to the diet of the recovering man at the appropriate time, and his metabolic rate, blood type, and/or ancestry dictate a need for it, he will deteriorate. Because of these factors, some men will do better on a maintenance diet of lean meats eaten more frequently; others will fare better on lighter proteins like fish and fowl eaten less often. Most should avoid dairy. All, I feel confident in saying, should incorporate some animal products, even if it's just a few eggs a week. Diets of healthy peoples around the world have been composed of highly nourishing traditional foods and devoid of junk food and empty calories, but they have all included some animal products. This was confirmed by Dr. Weston Price (himself a vegetarian) in his classic study of the diets of indigenous cultures in the early 1900s.

The healthy man may benefit from incorporating fresh vegetable juices into his diet on a routine basis and may even wish to use them exclusively for a day or two to cleanse his system and help replenish his alkaline mineral reserve. Such a mono-food diet, however, should not be extended beyond a few days because of the inherent lack of macronutrient balance.

## THE TRACE-MINERAL CONNECTION

Most people assimilate only a small percentage of the protein they take in, generally about 20 percent. Most people are also deficient in trace minerals needed for electrolyte formation. There is a relationship between the two previous statements. Read them again. **Trace minerals enable the body to use proteins.** By returning the needed minerals to our soils and our bodies, electrolyte balance would be reestablished. We would assimilate a greater percentage of the protein we eat and therefore need less of it. In the face of trace-mineral deficiency, homeostasis is disrupted due to electrolyte imbalance, body pH is thrown off, and digestion is impaired, limiting our ability to produce enzymes to break down protein and other nutrients. According to Gillian Martlew, N.D., author of *Electrolytes: The Spark of Life*:

> Filling up with protein or large amounts of separate amino acids unaccompanied by electrolytes saturates the body with harmful waste products. This is caused by the incomplete conversion of protein to amino acids. In this situation, the body creates uric acid instead of new tissue, and is then forced to use more minerals trying to neutralize it. . . . The enzymes needed for digestion are created from amino acids with the help of electrolytes. Minerals enable proteins to be broken down into their component parts (amino acids), which then become bioavailable—available for body use.[2]

Protein, then, is essentially useless and toxic to the body in the absence of electrolytes needed to produce the enzymes necessary to break it down into amino acids. It is highly recommended that all men include supplemental trace minerals in the form of a true-electrolyte formula (containing liquid minerals in crystalloid form) in their diet on a regular basis.

## DON'T FORGET

The important things to remember about protein are:

Balance it with other macronutrients (40/30/30, modified by considerations of ancestry, blood type, and metabolic rate).

Include some animal protein (amount to be determined by genetic and biochemical considerations).

Provide electrolytes in a usable form to ensure proper breakdown into amino acids.

# CHAPTER 5

# SUPER NUTRITION
# FOR THE PROSTATE

Prostate problems stem from genetic, hormonal, and dietary factors. While you may have no control over your genes, you do have control over your diet which, as we have seen, directly effects hormonal factors. When it comes to problems with the prostate, choosing "watchful waiting" and nutrition over aggressive medical treatments may be the best medicine of all.

One of the most powerful healing nutrients, the EFAs, are absolutely critical to the health of the prostate gland. By increasing the right fats (from nuts, seeds, and therapeutic oils) you can significantly support and nourish this vital gland and thereby decrease the chances of developing problems with it. The best initial medicine may be the essential fats, and avoidance of the non-essential, harmful trans fats from margarine, vegetable shortenings, fried foods, and processed vegetable oils.

The increase in trans-fat consumption over the past several decades can be correlated with a dramatic increase in prostate disorders. Harvard researchers Walter Willett and associates suggest there is a positive correlation between dietary intake of the trans fats and the rise of cancer. And shockingly, the culprit is not as much animal fats, as vegetable fats because statistics show that the consumption of animal fats has decreased by 30 percent since the beginning of the century, while vegetable-fat consumption is up 30 percent.

In addition, you've been told time and again that men who eat diets high in saturated fat—particularly red meat—have the greatest risk for prostate cancer. Well, that's just part of the story because what's missing from this advice is recognition of the critical role of the EFAs in balancing and regulating saturated fats.

We've already seen some of the ways in which hormonal output can be influenced by food. Prostate problems, brought on by a lifetime of bad eating, can be turned around by dietary changes that support the gland by reestablishing hormonal balance.

## STATISTICALLY SPEAKING

Prostate problems can occur at any time in your adult life, but the most common one, Benign prostatic hyperplasia (BPH), which is non-malignant enlargement of the prostate gland, primarily effects men over fifty. The incidence of the disorder increases with age: By age fifty, approximately 30 percent of all males in this country will begin to experience the symptoms of BPH. By sixty, half will be affected. Beyond the age of seventy, almost 80 percent will develop the disorder. And, by age eighty, almost every man in the U.S. will have BPH. It is the main problem treated by urologists. Some consider it to be a natural consequence of aging.

BPH can lead to cancer. An estimated 20 percent of those with BPH will develop prostate cancer. While prostate cancer was relatively rare before 1900, it is increasingly prevalent today. Like BPH, it is most common in the latter years. Only 2 percent of all prostate cancers occur in men under fifty. (Testicular cancer, on the other hand, is most common in the younger age groups, primarily affecting those between fifteen and thirty-four). In 1994, two hundred thousand cases of prostate cancer were diagnosed, with thirty-eight deaths resulting from it.

Younger men are not immune to prostate problems. Those between the ages of twenty and fifty may be prone to develop prostatitis, which is an inflammation, with or without infection, of the prostate gland.

## ABOUT THE PROSTATE

The prostate is a gland about the size of a walnut, located at the base of the bladder, surrounding both the urethra and the ejaculatory duct. This duct connects into the urethra and opens up into it. The prostate is an accessory sex gland that assists in the reproductive process by secreting an ejaculatory fluid that enhances the delivery and fertility of sperm. Secretion from the prostate gland constitutes about 80 percent of the fluid volume of semen. It receives sperm from the testicles, assists in the passage of that sperm and produces nutrients that nourish it. The prostate gland also serves to protect the genitourinary system against infection. The gland acts as a valve that permits both sperm and urine to flow in the proper direction.

During childhood, the prostate gland is quite small, just a little larger than a pencil eraser. Its growth and functioning are controlled by the male hormone, testosterone, which, at puberty facilitates not only prostate growth, but growth of sex organs and body hair, as well as change of voice. By age twenty, the prostate has achieved its full size, but after age forty it begins to enlarge. This growth is hormone induced.

While testosterone levels have begun to decline by this time of life, production of one of its metabolites, dihydrotestosterone (DHT), increases. It is this increase that is associated not only with prostate enlargement, but also with male pattern baldness. It appears that the aging process brings on both the decline of testosterone production and the increased conversion of testosterone to DHT. An increase in this conversion is what gives rise to growth of tissue in the prostate gland. This growth, unchecked, will ultimately lead to obstruction of the urethra, which passes through it.

## BENIGN PROSTATIC HYPERPLASIA

Benign prostatic hyperplasia (previously called benign prostatic hypertrophy) is the technical term for this hormone-mediated enlargement of the gland. The enzyme that converts testosterone to DHT is testosterone 5-alpha reductase. It is concentrated in the prostate, scrotal skin, testicles, and the scalp (hence the connection with male pattern baldness). DHT levels increase within prostate cells as a result of increased activity of this enzyme, as well as a greater uptake of testosterone and a lower rate of breakdown and excretion of DHT.

This leads to prostate enlargement, which results in urethral constriction and the development of BPH symptoms including weak stream of urine, dribbling, progressive frequency, urgency, hesitancy, and intermittency of urination. It is a condition that can be painful. Men with prostate enlargement often have to get up three to five times a night to urinate. In 2-3 percent of BPH cases, urinary incontinence results from instability of the detrusor muscle (the outer muscle layer of the bladder). Any man experiencing these symptoms is strongly urged to consult a physician for a definitive diagnosis. If left untreated, the condition can result in complete blockage of the bladder outlet, causing uremia (urine retention in the blood).

## TREATING BPH

Surgery is the most recommended treatment for BPH. There are three different surgical procedures utilized, but TransUrethral Resection of the Prostate (TURP) is the one performed on 95 percent of patients. Four hundred thousand of these procedures are done each year. It's the most common surgery performed on men over sixty-five. The TURP involves removal of the central core of the gland to take pressure off the urethra. A significant complication in this surgery is excessive absorption of irrigating fluid that produces what is known as "TURP Syndrome" characterized by "mental confusion with nausea and vomiting. It can lead to high blood pressure, heart failure, and seizures."[1] The surgery claims a 90 percent success rate, however:

> According to Dr. John Weinberg of Dartmouth Medical School, the death rate has been as high as 1.8 percent (one death per 56 procedures), 8 percent are hospitalized within three months because of complications, 5 percent (1 out of 20) become impotent, and about 20 percent (1 out of 5) will need another resection.[2]

In addition to TURP Syndrome, complications from this surgery include incontinence (temporary and, more rarely, permanent) and retrograde ejaculation (affecting $\frac{1}{2}$ or more of the patients) in which the man ejaculates backward into the bladder instead of into the penis.

A less invasive medical approach to treating early-stage prostate cancer involves a relatively new procedure in which radioactive pellets are implanted into the prostate gland. This procedure is done on an outpatient basis; it is therefore less costly than surgery and results in more rapid recovery and in fewer complications. One study, involving 298 prostate cancer patients found that 91 percent of those receiving the treatment were free of cancer five years later, compared to 82-89 percent of those treated surgically.

The drug considered to be most effective at controlling BPH symptoms acts by blocking the conversion of testosterone to DHT. The drug Finasteride (Proscar) accomplishes this by inhibiting the enzyme testosterone 5-alpha reductase. Proscar has been on the market for only about three years. It works slowly, taking approximately three months to accomplish maximum shrinkage (28 percent). It must be taken indefinitely and, like most drugs, has undesirable side-effects. These can include impotence and decreased libido. And, it is costly—several dollars per day. Even so, annual sales are expected to top one billion dollars this year. The cost of hospital care and surgery for BPH in the U.S. is also over one billion dollars per year. A less expensive, less invasive, safer, and more effective approach to BPH management may be found in nature's pharmacy.

## NATURE'S PHARMACY

Saw palmetto *(Serenoa repens)* is a small palm tree that grows along the Atlantic coast from South Carolina to Florida. An extract from its berries has proved to be an effective remedy for an enlarged prostate. This herb has been used for centuries by herbalists and American Indians to treat urinary tract problems and has also been considered by some to be a mild aphrodisiac. The French pioneered research in the clinical use of saw palmetto for BPH, establishing that its mode of action is the same as Proscar—it blocks the formation of DHT by inhibiting testosterone 5-alpha reductase. It has also been found to display other modes of action that prevent DHT uptake by the prostate cells and therefore is described by French scientists as a "multi-site inhibitor."

One double-blind study involving 110 BPH patients found after one month that the group using the herbal extract improved as follows: decreased nocturia (nightime urination) of more than 45 percent, increased urinary flow rate over 50 percent and reduced post-urination residual volume (the amount of urine retained in the bladder following urination) by 42 percent. By contrast, the placebo group showed only slight reduction in nocturia, no improvement in urine flow and actually increased in post-urinary residual volume. Ratings of outcome by physicians and patients both showed "significant" improvement in the group treated with saw palmetto, whereas this was not so for the placebo group.[3]

European research indicates that the greatest therapeutic benefits of the herb are found in the fat and sterol portions of the plant. This finding gave rise to the production of a standardized extract of the fat-soluble (liposterolic) fraction of saw palmetto berries. There are many types of saw palmetto preparations on the market and some are more potent than others, as the chart below indicates:

| Types of Saw Palmetto | Relative strength to 85-95% extract |
|---|---|
| Dried berry | 5% |
| Liquid tincture extract | 5–10% |
| Powdered extract 4:1 | 25% |
| Liquid oil 10:1 extract | 50% |
| Liquid oil 20:1 85-95% extract | 100% |

It is the last item, the liquid oil 20:1 that is the form used in the European clinical studies. It contains 85-95 percent sterols and fatty acids and, in the studies, was given in amounts averaging 320 mg. per day. The program I have developed (see Appendix B), includes the most potent extract of saw palmetto.

Treating prostate disease with saw palmetto extract has not only been proven to be extremely effective, but it costs less than a third as much as prescription remedies, and is safer. Between 1983 and 1992, nine double-blind studies conducted involving 528 BPH patients have concluded that the extract of saw palmetto was effective. The conclusion based upon both objective and subjective measurements of prostate enlargement. **And**, all studies demonstrated no toxicity.

## NUTRITIONAL AND HERBAL SUPPORT

Inadequate diet appears to be a primary factor in the development of BPH. For this reason, it usually responds to nutritional and herbal support, especially in the early stages. The extent of dietary advice that most doctors are likely to dispensed is apt to be limited to the recommendation that spices, alcohol, caffeine, and other irritating foods be avoided and that the fluid intake be kept high. This is good advice, but there's more to know and to do.

Perhaps the most important element in a nutritional program to prevent/treat BPH is the trace mineral, zinc. Zinc deficiency is common today, for the mineral is deficient in the soils of thirty-two states. It is removed in processing and is depleted by smoking, alcohol, coffee, infections, and medications. The ability to absorb zinc declines with age. A normal prostate gland contains more zinc than any other organ in the body. Because the prostate serves as a storehouse, some believe that when zinc is needed elsewhere, the body robs the prostate, thus depriving it of this critically important trace element.

As previously mentioned, zinc (as well as $B_6$) plays an important role in many aspects of hormonal metabolism. It is perhaps for this reason that it is effective in reducing prostate size and symptoms. Good sources of zinc include seafood (especially oysters), organ meats, soybeans, meat, eggs, brewer's yeast, and seeds. Both $B_6$ and zinc play an important role in nourishing the prostate gland.

Other nutrients important to prostate health include vitamins C and E and the mineral selenium. These are all antioxidant nutrients, generally deficient in the SAD, and needed to offset free radical damage to cells and preserve oxygen. Another antioxidant-potent nutrient used for prostate problems is pycnogenol from pine bark and grape seed. These extracts are rich a source of substances called anthocyanidins and proanthocyanidins, flavonoids (pigments) that have exceptionally powerful antioxidant effects.

Extra amounts of B vitamins will help the body to deal with the stress of any illness, including BPH. Stress increases the need for this family of vitamins. Increased intake of vitamin A will help prevent and/or resolve infection. Beta-carotene, a precursor of vitamin A can be used as well.

Adding nuts and seeds to the diet, or increasing the intake of them, is a tasty way to provide an extra source of both zinc and the EFAs. Lack of these good fats seems to be a major factor in development of BPH. So, increasing the intake of EFA-rich oils from various nuts, as well as flax seed and evening primrose oils has a regulating effect on the saturated animal fats in the diet. It's not simply a matter of decreasing animal fat and protein, as has been generally recommended, but balancing the total fat intake with the good fat.

Prostatic and seminal lipid (fat) levels and ratios are often abnormal in BPH and significant improvement can be attained by administering an EFA complex containing linoleic and linolenic acids.[4] It would appear that a prostaglandin deficiency may be a cause of BPH. Since

EFAs are precursors to prostaglandins, they are vital to normal prostate function.

Pumpkin seeds are a rich source of both EFAs and zinc. So, the folklore medicine remedy of eating $\frac{1}{4}$ to $\frac{1}{2}$ cup of these seeds daily for prostate problems may indeed have value. Pumpkin seed oil, found in most health food stores, may also be used. In addition, remember that a high-carbohydrate diet should be avoided and all forms of sugar (including fruit, fruit juice, and sweeteners) severely limited, because they stress the hormonal and immune systems.

If you suffer from BPH, you may also benefit from taking a glandular extract (protomorphogen) of prostate tissue. These are produced from bovine (cow) and porcine (pig) sources. Raw glandular concentrates appear to provide the template, or pattern, from which the body can build new cells. Healthy bovine or porcine prostate extract ingested by a man with prostate enlargement, is more beneficial, it seems, than actually eating the organ meat would be. After being refined, raw glandular tissue assumes an enzyme-like action that improves assimilation by the target organ, in this case the prostate.

It has been found that exposure to cadmium (from cigarette smoke, paints, contaminated drinking water, shellfish found near industrial shores, etc.) will stimulate the growth of human prostatic tissue and that proper concentrations of the mineral, selenium will inhibit that growth.[5] Those men with BPH will want to rule out cadmium toxicity. This can be done through hair analysis.

Amino acids can also be used to treat BPH. One study indicates that supplementation with a combination of L-glutamic acid, L-alanine, and glycine (two 6-grain caps taken three times daily for two weeks, followed by one cap taken three times daily) may be beneficial. The study, involving forty-five patients supplemented with this combination of amino acids, showed reduction or relief of nocturia in 95 percent of the cases, urgency reduced in 81 percent, frequency reduced in 73 percent, and delayed urination in 70 percent.[6]

Another factor to consider is when lactobacillus in the body are deficient, prostate trouble, as well as hair loss and abnormal fat distribution can result. Supplements of acidophilus bacteria can therefore be helpful. Bear in mind, however, that these beneficial bacteria will not grow in the intestines unless the body pH is near perfect—and pH is regulated by our old friends, the electrolytes. So you'll want to add them to your supplemental regimen.

In addition to saw palmetto, the powdered bark of the *Pygeum africanus* tree, has been useful in the treatment of BPH. It has been used for centuries as a treatment for urinary disorders and has been found by French scientists to have anti-inflammatory properties and no toxic side-effects, even in large doses and with prolonged use. Clinical trials have shown its efficacy in alleviating symptoms. Another herb useful in this regard is *Aletrius farinosa* (Star Grass). Stinging nettle is also recommended by herbalists for BPH.

## PROSTATITIS

Prostatitis, as mentioned, is most common in men under fifty and involves inflammation or infection of the prostate gland. The infectious variety can be either acute or chronic and is associated with a pathogen, such as a bacteria or chlamydia (a sexually transmitted parasite). When there is a deficiency of glandular elements such as zinc, vitamin C, and proteolytic enzymes (enzymes that break down proteins), favorable conditions are established for infection to develop. The glandular elements can be depleted as a result of excessive consumption of caffeine, alcohol, and spicy foods, which leads to lowered immunity. Increased sexual activity can lead to the development of prostatitis, for it depletes the prostate gland of enzymes and zinc, nutrients that sterilize the urethra and protect the gland from infection.

Symptoms of acute prostatitis include difficult urination characterized by frequency, urgency, and a burning sensation during urination, as well as a discharge from the penis following bowel movements. Prostatic pain and tenderness, which can extend into the pelvis and back, can be present in the beginning of an acute infection and may be followed by fever, chills, and generalized fatigue.

Symptoms of chronic infection are similar, but not as severe. Because of their mildness, these symptoms may be ignored by some men. This is not wise, however, for left untreated, a chronic infection of the prostate can result in infection in the kidney or epididymis (a tube along the back of the testicles), as well as swollen, painful testicles (orchitis), bladder outlet obstruction, and prostate stones.

Non-bacterial prostatitis is the most common type. The symptoms are the same as for bacterial prostatitis, but no infectious agent is located, though white cells are present in prostatic fluid, a sign of inflammation. The cause of this condition is unknown. Both types of prostatitis are commonly treated with antibiotics—short-term for acute and long-term for chronic. The non-bacterial type may also be treated with prostate massage, hot baths, antispasmodics, tranquilizers, and anti-inflammatory medication.

Another type of prostatitis, known as prostatodynia, involves essentially the same symptoms as described above, but no abnormalities are found on examination or in the urinalysis. This condition is thought to be due to muscle spasms and is generally treated with medication and hot baths.

Herbal preparations may be useful in the treatment of prostatitis. An evergreen plant known as pipsissewa (*Chimaphilia umbellata*), is useful for chronic infectious prostatitis, as well as other urinary disorders. It contains a powerful antiseptic, arbutin, which helps nourish the urinary tract and prostate and increase blood flow to them. Arbutin is also the active ingredient in uva ursi, another herb that is beneficial to the urinary tract.

Horsetail, a rich source of the trace element, silica, may be useful in the treatment of acute prostatic infection. An herb that assists in fighting any type of infection, including prostatitis, is *Echinacea angustifolia*. Garlic also has natural antibiotic properties. Other herbs that may be useful for decreasing pain, irritation, swelling, and impotence associated with prostatitis include: *Delphinia staphysagria*, *Thuja occidentalis*, and *Anemone pulsatilla*. These herbs are frequently administered in homeopathic form (a homeopathic preparation is prepared through the dilution and potentiation of a small amount of the herb that becomes energized through the process).

Supplementation with vitamins, minerals, and EFAs as outlined for BPH is recommended, emphasizing increased intake of vitamins A and C where infection is present. Extra amounts of calcium and magnesium can help relax muscles.

## PROSTATE CANCER

Prostate cancer is known as a "silent cancer" because few symptoms are usually felt initially. As the tumor grows it tends to constrict the urethra and present the same symptoms as BPH. It has been noted that BPH can lead to prostate cancer and that its onset generally occurs in the latter years of life. In fact, the average man, at the time he is diagnosed with prostate cancer is seventy-three years old. One out of every eight men will develop prostate cancer in his lifetime.

The prostate is one of four sites in the body that account for more than half of all cancer deaths. The other three are lungs, colon, and breast. While breast cancer is infrequent in men, lung cancer is the number one killer, prostate is second, and colon and rectum cancer run a close third.

Because its onset is usually late in life and because it is most often a slow-growing cancer, it has been argued that "watchful waiting" should take preference over aggressive treatment. Many men die of other causes before prostate cancer creates any real problem, and medical treatment (surgery and radiation) can produce complications (loss of bladder control, impotence, and rectal injury). According to autopsies, over half of all men over the age of fifty have cancerous prostate cells, but only 2.4 percent eventually die of the disease. Many men with prostate cancer, unaware of its existence, die of an unrelated cause. The cancer isn't discovered until an autopsy reveals its presence.

For these reasons, some view early detection of this cancer as a questionable benefit. There are no studies showing that early screening for prostate cancer can actually save lives, and the death rate for the cancer has remained pretty much unchanged for decades, despite advances in medicine. Techniques used for diagnosis include Digital Rectal Exam (DRE), blood tests, tissue biopsy, and a number of visualization techniques such as x-ray, MRI, ultrasound, and CT scan that provide an image of the structures inside the body.

In the DRE, the physician will perform a rectal exam, feeling the prostate through the wall of the rectum. Hardness indicates a possible cancer (though may also be a sign of infection or stones). The DRE may be normal even when cancer is present, though this is unlikely. The American Cancer Society recommends annual DRE examination for all men over forty.

A commonly used blood test for diagnosing cancer is the Prostate-Specific Antigen Test (PSA). This test was developed in 1989. In its first year of use, it increased the number of diagnosed cases of prostate cancer by 16 percent. Even before that, diagnosis—and subsequently treatment—was increasing. From 1984 to 1990, surgical removal of cancerous prostates in men sixty-five and over increased 500-600 percent.

The PSA test is used to detect or confirm both BPH and cancer. PSA is a protein substance unique to the prostate. It is slightly elevated in BPH and greatly increased in prostate cancer. Infection can also cause elevation of PSA levels. The higher the PSA level, the greater the chance of metastasis (spreading to other parts of the body). When prostate cancer spreads, three-quarters of the time it spreads to bone. Some men do not seek medical attention until they experience fatigue, weight loss, and bone pain, symptoms of wide-spread disease.

Nutritional advocate, Julian Whitaker, M.D., voiced concern in the November, 1994 edition of his newsletter, *Health and Healing*, that the increasing use of PSA screening will lead to increased use of surgery, radiation, and chemotherapy, which they have. These treatments have the potential of doing harm. He points to a study done in the *Journal of the American Medical Association*, which concluded that neither early detection, nor conventional treatment of prostate cancer, resulted in a significant extension of life span. They did, in fact, reduce the quality of the patient's remaining years, due to such adverse side-effects as impotency.

Dr. Whitaker states that, in his own practice, he uses the PSA test in a different way—as a barometer of the success of nutritional treatment that includes saw palmetto and dietary changes. The power of conservative nutritional regimens is reflected in dropping PSA levels, witnessed many times by Dr. Whitaker.

I personally would suggest that more physicians should take the Whitaker approach. I encourage all of my male patients in their early forties and fifties to start on saw palmetto as soon as possible, along with banishing trans fats from their lives forever.

You see, PSA results are not as clear-cut as one would hope. In 1993 it was reported that approximately 40 percent of men with prostate cancer show up negative; of those that have no symptoms, but a positive PSA, only one out of 75 to 150 actually do have cancer, and false positives occur in one out of four men with symptoms. These statistics refer to the **standard** PSA test. A new PSA test has recently been developed that is said to be more reliable. A problem with false positives is that the suspicious results will generally prompt a biopsy, which carries with it some risk; therefore, it is desirable to reduce the number of "low yield" prostate biopsies being performed. Steps are being taken in this direction and a sixteen-year study—designed to resolve the controversy as to whether early screening, detection, and treatment actually does extend the lives of men with prostate cancer—is now underway.

The American Cancer Society recommends annual PSA tests for all men fifty and over. They also recommend that high-risk men be tested annually beginning at age forty. High-risk men include those with a family history of prostate cancer and African-Americans. Based on new studies, we can add men who have had vasectomies to the list. The problem with vasectomies is this: As sperm builds up in the sealed-off vas deferens, it is re-absorbed by the body, which reacts by launching an auto-immune response to its own tissue.

African-American men have the highest incidence in the world of prostate cancer. Their risk of developing it is 40 percent greater than it is for whites. The interesting thing is that, while **American** blacks have a death rate from prostate cancer that is almost double that of whites, the incidence of the cancer in **Nigerian** blacks is only one-sixth that of U.S. blacks. Another interesting fact is that, while prostate cancer death rate in Japan is only one-seventh of ours, when Japanese men relocate to the U.S., their prostate cancer rate rapidly increases.

## THE DIETARY CONNECTION

These statistics point to a cultural factor influencing the development of prostate cancer, one that overrides genetic influences. That factor involves lifestyle and diet. Our men typically lead a stressful, fast-paced life, are exposed to environmental toxins, and regularly consume a diet of devitalized, processed junk food. Please remember that prostate cancer was relatively rare before 1900—that is, before the advent of food processing, the widespread use of pesticides, and other environmental toxins, and the fat-free, high-carbohydrate diet.

A major difference in diet with regard to the above referenced cultures is this: The Japanese and Nigerians eat much less animal fat and many more vegetables than we do. Numerous studies have indicated that the nutrients and anutrients (fiber, pigments, and phytochemicals) in vegetables have a protective effect against cancer and, of course, we've all heard of the link between heavy meat consumption and cancer. A 1993 Harvard School of Public Health Study found that men who eat red meat five times a week are 2.6 times more likely to develop advanced, often fatal, prostate cancer than are men who eat red meat one time or less.[7] The balanced use of essential fats in the diet would probably change this situation dramatically.

Though a source of saturated fat, meat of itself is not a bad food. Meat from organically raised animals, eaten by a healthy man whose intake of EFAs, fiber, vitamins, minerals, and other nutrients is adequate can be an excellent source of vitally needed protein. However, a man with cancer is not healthy. For him, excessive consumption of meat—especially without the addition of Omega-3 EFAs from such oils as fish and flax seed—will create conditions of further imbalance. Being out of balance (homeostasis), his body lacks the trace minerals (to form electrolytes) that must be present to produce enzymes necessary for break down of protein into amino acids. Additionally, the hydrochloric acid needed for protein digestion declines with age and will, most likely, be inadequate in the middle-aged or older man with prostate cancer.

Supplements of HCl and proteolytic enzymes can be helpful to support the digestive process until it can be normalized by the restoration of electrolyte balance through the regular use of Trace-Lyte in combination with a balanced diet.

## EAT YOUR VEGGIES

Italian and Swiss researchers compared 8,077 people with 19 different types of cancer with 6,147 people without cancer. They were each divided into three different groups: Those who ate less than seven vegetables per week, those who ate seven per week, and those who ate more than seven per week. They found that a man who eats seven servings of vegetables per week has 20 percent less risk of developing prostate cancer than one who eats fewer than seven. And, a man who eats more than seven servings has a 70 percent less chance than one who eats less than seven. Seven vegetables per week is only one per day, and yet, even that small amount confers some protection. We should at least triple that amount.

The National Institute of Cancer recommends that Americans consume a minimum of three to five servings of vegetables daily. Most Americans, especially men, fall quite short of this, even though a serving is only half a cup. Vegetables provide a wide range of nutrients and anutrients. They are a source, not only of vitamins and minerals, but also of carbohydrates and protein. Among plant pigments are carotenes, flavonoids, and chlorophyll. Beta is just one of over 400 carotenes. All have potent antioxidant and anticancer effects.

Tissue carotene content can be increased by juicing a wide variety of vegetables, a practice highly recommended for cancer patients. The nutrients in freshly prepared juices are concentrated and are easily used by the body. Flavonoids provide protection from free-radical damage. They are found largely in fruits and flowers. Pycnogenol and grape seed extract are part of this group. They have extremely powerful antioxidant activity. Chlorophyll, the green plant pigment, has also been shown to have significant antioxidant and anti-cancer effects.

Vegetables are best consumed in their fresh state. Use frozen in preference to canned if fresh is not available and select organic whenever possible. If commercially grown vegetables are used, wash or soak them first in a 3 percent hydrogen peroxide solution (preferably food grade) to remove pesticides, mold, and bacteria. A diluted Clorox solution may also be used, but only with purified water, as the pollutants in water will unite with chlorine to form potentially carcinogenic compounds. Using the Clorox bath has the added benefit of killing parasites (a growing health hazard discussed in Chapter 12). To prepare a Clorox bath, add a half teaspoon of bleach to a gallon of purified or distilled water. Soak food for 15-30 minutes, then soak in clear water for 10 minutes.

Vegetables should not be overcooked, as this destroys important nutrients. The best cooking methods are light steaming, baking, or quick stir frying. Never boil vegetables, unless they're being made into soup.

One vegetable in particular, the Japanese maitake mushroom, has shown promise in treating prostate, as well as other cancers. Naturopathic physician, Peter D'Adamo, editor of the *Journal of Naturopathic Medicine* has reported success in his private practice in Greenwich, Connecticut, using maitake to treat men with prostate cancer in whom chemotherapy has been unsuccessful. The mushroom has also been used with success by Dr. D'Adamo in treating pulmonary metastasis (where the cancer has spread through the lungs and circulatory system) and cancers of the liver, breast, and colon. Others have reported that maitake helps combat chronic fatigue syndrome, high blood pressure, diabetes, and HIV.

Abraham Ber, M.D., a homeopathic physician who practices orthomolecular medicine in Phoenix, Arizona, also reports success with using the maitake mushroom in his practice over a two-year period. He has treated at least a dozen prostate cancer patients with maitake tablets and obtained encouraging results, including improved urinary flow and decreased frequency.

These mushrooms have a powerful strengthening effect on the immune system. Maitake is considered to be an adaptogen. As such, it assists the body in adapting to any form of stress and helps regulate endocrine activity and other body functions to achieve balance or homeostasis. It has recently been found that maitake mushrooms taken by patients undergoing standard chemotherapy reduced the amount of chemotherapy drugs needed by 50 percent without compromising the anti-cancer results of the treatment.

Recent findings, based on a study conducted at Memorial Sloan-Kettering Cancer Center in New York, indicate that men who regularly consumed the common spice, cumin, had a significantly lower rate of urological cancers (including prostate cancer) than those who consumed little of the spice.

Joe was a fifty-five-year-old contractor who sought my services after being diagnosed with prostate cancer. He had decided not to go the "traditional" route with chemotherapy and wanted to discuss the watchful waiting approach. After reviewing his chart and assessing his dietary history, we drew up a dietary regimen with herbal support.

My first recommendation was to eliminate **all** trans fats from his diet. Joe's love affair with MacDonald's French fries was over. I strongly suggested that he cut back on his meat consumption and only use sources that were organic. Increasing his zinc and essential fatty acids intake was accomplished with the addition of nuts and seeds (specifically pumpkin seeds) to his diet. I also recommended that he supplement with evening primrose and flax oils, and additional zinc as well. Supplemental saw palmetto and antioxidant nutrients including pycnogenol, vitamins C, and E, and the mineral selenium were included in his treatment plan as well as maitake mushroom extract. Joe felt strongly that he could always resort to chemotherapy if he needed it. So far, so good.

## ENVIRONMENTAL FACTORS

There is an established link between pesticide use and cancer. Our crops are treated with 1.2 billion pounds of pesticides and herbicides yearly. Studies have shown that farmers run a higher risk of developing certain cancers, including cancer of the prostate.[8] Over 600 pesticides are currently used in the U.S. The Environmental Protection Agency has identified 64 of them as potentially cancer-causing. The EPA sets tolerance levels for pesticides in raw and unprocessed foods. The FDA is responsible for enforcing the levels set by the EPA. However, they do not test for all pesticides and actually screen only a very small percentage of our food supply (probably less than one percent). In addition, foods that are found to exceed the legal limits of pesticide residues are not prevented from going to market!

Imported produce has perhaps twice the level of pesticide residue that domestic food has and should be avoided. Pesticides banned in this country are often exported to other countries that use them on their crops and then import them back to us! In addition to washing or soaking produce to remove pesticide residues, it is wise to assure a high intake of fiber (chiefly from vegetables) and antioxidants (vitamins A, C, and E and the minerals selenium and zinc) in the diet to help eliminate pesticides from the body.

In addition to avoiding pesticide residues in food, you will also want to avoid environmental exposure to chemicals. Instead of using chemical pesticides to rid your home of roaches and fleas, use natural alternatives or call in a natural pest control service. And, instead of using chemical fertilizers on your lawn, use organic ones.

The man with prostate cancer will, of course, want to avoid smoking and avoid exposure to second hand smoke, as well. Cigarette smoke is a major source of cadmium toxicity. Studies show that cadmium may promote cancer by replacing zinc in the prostate.[9]

Exposure to ElectroMagnetic Fields (EMFs) appears to be another factor in the development of prostate cancer. Studies show that EMFs can suppress the pineal gland's secretion of the hormone, melatonin. It is the suppression of this function that has been implicated in the etiology of prostate cancer. Melatonin plays a key role in preventing and reversing cancer. It increases the cytotoxicity of the body's natural killer lymphocytes, thereby inhibiting tumor growth. It will therefore be important to limit exposure to EMFs as much as possible by keeping electrical appliance use to a minimum in your home.*

Another environmental factor that affects the likelihood of developing cancer has to do with exposure to sunlight. If you're thinking that such exposure increases the risk, you've got it backwards. The sun converts cholesterol on our skin to vitamin D. Duke University researchers have found that this vitamin is protective against prostate cancer. A University of North Carolina study showed that men living in the northern latitudes, with less exposure to the ultraviolet rays of the sun are at greater risk for developing prostate cancer.

John Ott has done a great deal of research on the beneficial effects of sunlight. To reap its benefits, we must take in the rays—all of them, including UV—through the retina of our eyes. Spending time (at least half an hour) outside (even in the shade) without glasses or sunglasses

---

*For further information on the detrimental effects of EMFs and how to avoid or reduce them, contact the Baubiologie Institute at 813-461-4371.

(which block UV) can therefore be an important part of a prevention or recovery program.

## PUTTING IT TOGETHER

Since prostate cancer symptoms are, for the most part, identical to BPH symptoms, all of the nutritional advice given for BPH applies to prostate cancer as well. Since those with BPH may later develop prostate cancer, they may want to incorporate some of the nutritional advice given in this chapter for that condition. While zinc levels are low in BPH patients, they're even lower in those with prostate cancer. So, zinc supplementation becomes especially important for males with prostate cancer.

One large, ten-year study involving 2,440 men, ages fifty and older, showed an inverse relationship between serum vitamin A and prostate cancer incidence. The men who developed the cancer had significantly lower vitamin A levels than those who did not develop it.[10]

In using herbs for prostate cancer, know that they are not specific for the different types of tumors, but act rather as overall immune system stimulants. In addition to the herbs mentioned in the BPH section, the following can help treat prostate cancer: poke weed, mistletoe, meadow saffron, foxglove, poison hemlock, and burdock. Other immune-enhancing herbs that may be useful include: pau d'arco, ginseng, licorice root, and golden seal. Additionally, CoQ10 and Royal Jelly will assist in building immunity and strength in both men with prostate cancer and those with BPH. See the next chapter for a discussion of CoQ10. Royal Jelly is a salivary secretion of honeybees that is rich in amino acids, B vitamins and other nutrients. It has been used to support functioning of the sex organs and to treat sterility. Adding the cruciferous vegetables, such as broccoli and cauliflower and other green and orange vegetables to the diet can also help. See Appendix B for specific supplement guidelines for cancer and other prostate problems.

## GET THAT CHECK UP

Remember to have a rectal exam yearly after the age of forty, as well as an annual PSA after age fifty (forty if you're high risk). But remember the PSA may not be definitive. Additionally, see your doctor if any of these symptoms develop:

Lumps in the prostate and testicles
Thickening or excess fluid retention in the scrotum
Painful, weak, interrupted urination
Unexplained, persistent low back and leg pain

## POINTS TO REMEMBER

While testosterone production decreases with age, its conversion to DHT increases, giving rise to prostate problems and male pattern baldness.

While genetics plays a role in the development of prostate cancer, diet and lifestyle seem to have more bearing—and these are the factors that you can control.

Nutritional and herbal therapies can help prevent and treat prostate problems. Avoidance of sugar, damaged fats, processed foods, and the use of key elements such as antioxidant nutrients and especially the mineral zinc and herbs such as saw palmetto and the food spice, cumin, can be particularly beneficial.

# CHAPTER 6

# SUPER NUTRITION FOR
# THE MALE HEART

According to Dr. Bruce West: "The heart is the one organ of the body that is most easily influenced and healed with nutrition."[1] And in the past three decades we have been bombarded with nutritional information and dietary mandates that should have American hearts beating to a healthy beat. But this is not the case.

We as a nation are eating less meat and dietary cholesterol, smoking less cigarettes, and exercising more, but the incidence of heart disease has **increased** over the last fifteen years. And while the overall death rate from heart disease actually declined by 40 percent during that time, it still remains the leading cause of death in the U.S., and the leading cause of early death in men. By age sixty, one in every five men have suffered a heart attack.

More than 350,000 men will die of heart attacks this year.

All of the research and study done on cardiovascular disease seems to have produced a nation of confused, cardiac cripples. Sorting through the daily barrage of "heart smart" information from newspapers, magazines, radio, and television can be overwhelming. Certainly we all know that smoking, excess weight, lack of exercise, and poor eating habits are known risk factors for this fatal disease. And many of us still believe that consumption of dietary cholesterol and saturated fats are the leading cause of clogged arteries. We were told that switching from butter to margarine, from real eggs to Egg Beaters, was the wise thing to do.

But now we are being told that we were misinformed. That margarine is indeed bad for the cardiovascular system, and real eggs don't raise our cholesterol levels. And that cholesterol may not be the villain it has been portrayed as. I am reminded of a poem by James Kavanaugh that says that after listening to all the conflicting advice from numerous nutritionists and doctors, he decided it was just easier to live on fritos and Jack Daniels.

But hold those fritos and that Jack Daniels until you read this chapter. It will assist you in sorting through the newest information on risk factors and help you understand the role of cholesterol, sugar, insulin, drugs, our toxic environment, and iron overload in the development and progression of heart disease.

## CHOLESTEROL—FRIEND OR FOE?

Heart disease results when blood flow through coronary arteries (which supply the heart with oxygen and nutrients) becomes restricted or blocked. This causes damage to the heart muscle that results in a heart attack. Often—but not always—heart attacks result from atherosclerosis (hardening of the arteries), a condition where plaque (containing cholesterol and other materials) builds up in the arteries. Atherosclerosis is a degenerative condition affecting many people in our country, even the young. A 1993 study based on autopsies of 1,532 teenagers and young adults found that all of them had fatty patches in their aortas and 59 percent had heart disease.

It has become popular to blame cholesterol for all heart problems and to avoid cholesterol-containing food in an effort to prevent or treat the problem. There are many holes in this theory. Without question cholesterol has been associated with heart disease. Mosquitos have been associated with stagnant water. But mosquitos do not cause water to be stagnant any more than cholesterol causes plaque to build up in the arteries. Many feel that cholesterol deposits actually result from the body's efforts to repair arterial damage.

Cholesterol enters our body through dietary sources (from animal products such as meat and eggs). The body, however, also produces its own. That's right: The waxy, fat-like substance is produced in our own bodies, 80 percent of it manufactured in the liver and brain. It's contained in nearly every cell. Our bodies produce cholesterol because it is vitally needed to maintain our health. Consider these major functions:

Construction of cell walls
Production of male and female hormones
Production of adrenal hormones (like cortisone, released due to stress)
Production of bile acids (which break up fats for absorption)
Vitamin D synthesis (sunlight turns cholesterol into vitamin D)
Insulation of nerve fibers
Cell membrane repair

Cholesterol also has antioxidant properties, helping to fight disease-causing free radicals.

Deficiency of cholesterol has been associated with a number of conditions, including anemia, acute infection, excess thyroid function, autoimmune disorders, and cancer. The fact is that drugs which artificially lower cholesterol cause a number of cancers. When it comes to cholesterol, too little can be as much of a problem as too much. Once again, balance is the key.

The following chart of causes of high and low cholesterol was compiled by Dr. Cass Igram (*PPNF Nutritional Journal*, Vol 15, #1-2, 1991):

## CAUSES OF HIGH CHOLESTEROL LEVEL
excess **dietary sugar**
excess **dietary starch**
excess **hydrogenated or processed fats**
liver dysfunction
amino acid deficiency
EFA deficiency
deficiency of natural anti-oxidants
increased tissue damage due to infection, radiation, free radicals
alcoholism
food allergies

## CAUSES OF LOW CHOLESTEROL
immune decline
chronic hepatitis
cholesterol-lowering drugs
EFA deficiency
liver infection or disease
manganese deficiency
adrenal stress
street drugs

Cholesterol is actually a lubricant that is meant to keep the blood oily so that it can flow freely through the vessels. However, when inorganic mineral deposits collect on artery walls, cholesterol may adhere to them. Minerals tend to go out of solution and form deposits (in arteries and elsewhere) when the body's pH is out of balance. PH, you'll recall, is regulated by electrolytes. Certain trace minerals, because of their electrolyte activity, not only assure that minerals are kept in solution, but they also encourage proper liver function and improve digestion and metabolism of fats.

## THE ROLE OF THE LIVER

Liver function is critically important in cholesterol metabolism. The liver not only produces cholesterol, but also converts it into bile, and regulates its level in the blood. The properly functioning liver will adjust cholesterol production according to dietary intake, decreasing or increasing it as needed.

Eighty percent of the body's cholesterol is used in bile production. That bile, along with excess cholesterol, is stored in the gall bladder. When fat is present in the intestines, the gall bladder contracts, sending bile to the intestines to break down the fat. The bile is absorbed by the body in direct proportion to the amount of time it takes to pass out of the digestive tract.

Slow transit times, resulting from constipation, cause an excessive amount of bile to be reabsorbed. When bile is reabsorbed and recycled, less new bile is formed in the liver and cholesterol cannot be turned into bile at the same rate. Therefore, excessive cholesterol builds up. This theory was put forth by Dr. William Welles in his book *The Shocking Truth About Cholesterol* (1990). He states: "The real issue is bile flow, not diet."[2] One of the reasons that high-fiber foods, like oat bran, are effective in lowering cholesterol is that they decrease the reabsorption of bile salts and relieve constipation. From this perspective, factors like liver congestion and constipation, are a cause in the build-up of cholesterol.

I have found—almost without fail—that men with good elimination and healthy livers, can properly handle dietary cholesterol, as long as they are getting the nutrients necessary to metabolize it. I recommend a basic foundation for every heart smart nutrition plan that includes the EFAs, the minerals chromium and magnesium, and the B vitamins, niacin and choline. These elements are largely lacking in the SAD, and the incidence of liver dysfunction and constipation is high in our culture.

Because of faulty nutrution many people are not well able to handle the cholesterol in animal foods. This does not mean, however, that they should avoid cholesterol-containing foods. What it **does** mean, is that they should perhaps limit them, until balance is restored in the body. In an imbalanced state, neither the protein, nor the fat from animal products is properly metabolized. The thing to eliminate is not the fat, nor the protein, but rather the conditions of imbalance. This calls for elimination of processed, fragmented foods and restoration of essential nutrients, especially electrolytes.

## WHAT CHOLESTEROL LEVELS MEAN

The Framingham study, in progress for more than thirty years, was designed to investigate the risk factors in heart disease. The researchers have found that the level of cholesterol in the blood does correlate with heart disease. But there is no correlation found between cholesterol in the diet and heart disease. No significant differences in the blood cholesterol of people who ate several eggs per week (up to twenty-four) and those who ate only a few (up to two and a half).

The latest guidelines that we've been given about cholesterol levels is that total cholesterol should be less than 200 and HDL (the "good" cholesterol) should be greater than 35. Let's look at what HDL and LDL mean. Blood cholesterol does not travel through the body on its own, but must attach itself to a solid substance. In the bloodstream it binds with lipoproteins which, like cholesterol, are formed in the liver. HDL, high-density lipoprotein, has less cholesterol, more protein. It is composed principally of lecithin. Its job is to pull cholesterol back from body tissues to the liver where it's converted to bile and excreted. LDL stands for low-density lipoprotein. It carries cholesterol from the liver to parts of the body where it is needed.

The higher the HDL in relationship to total overall cholesterol, the lower the risk of heart disease. The ration between total cholesterol and HDL cholesterol is now considered more important than just the total cholesterol alone. Optimally, the ratio of total cholesterol to HDL should be 3:1.

I remember how anxious one of my clients was when he got his most recent blood test results. Peter was a forty-five-year-old mechanic with a history of heart disease in the family. His total cholesterol was a little over 200. When I asked him what the HDL was, he said 60. I quickly put his mind at ease and congratulated him on his heart-healthy ratio.

## FACTORS THAT AFFECT CHOLESTEROL LEVELS

### Good Fats and Bad Fats

A lack of the nutrients needed for cholesterol metabolism, paired with a deficiency of antioxidant nutrients are primary factors in the development of heart disease. The antioxidant nutrients—vitamins A, C, and E, selenium, and zinc—prevent oxidation of cholesterol. Foods left out at room temperature or those that are fried, smoked, cured, or aged become oxidized. They give rise to free radicals, renegade molecules, which damage blood vessel walls. The body then tries to repair the damage with cholesterol.

All processed foods, powdered milk, powdered eggs, dried custard mixes, cake mixes, aged cheeses, and smoked, dried, and aged meats, including bacon, ham, sausage, and packaged sandwich meats create free radicals. These foods can contribute significantly to the clogging of arteries.[3] It is important to understand that while powdered eggs are to be avoided, fresh ones can be included in the diet, as long as you don't fry them. Soft or hard boiled and poached are the best cooking methods.

As I have previously discussed, one of the most critical problems with the SAD is its lack of sufficient essential fatty acids. Both the Omega-3 and Omega-6 families of EFAs are involved in the regulation of cholesterol and triglycerides (blood fat) in the body and in the formation of many hormones. You'll recall that the higher the ratio of Omega-3s to Omega-6s, the less likely that a clot will obstruct an artery. Because of food processing and food choices, Omega-3s are in short supply in our diet. More are needed, especially the EPA form, through the intake of cold water fish, fish oils, and flax seed and canola oils, to regulate cholesterol.

Refined oils and man-made hydrogenated ones need to be **totally** eliminated from the diet, for the trans fats they form interfere with the functioning of EFAs and increase serum cholesterol. TFAs actually raise LDL, the "bad" cholesterol, and lower HDL, the "good." When Northern Europe's supply of hydrogenated foods was cut off during the last world war, the result was the most dramatic decline in heart disease of the century!

## Insulin Strikes Again

I have told you about the hormonal effects of food. The insulin response from a diet too high in carbohydrates produces "bad" eicosanoids that can lead to high blood pressure, heart attack, atherosclerosis, increased fat storage, unstable sugar levels, and more. You learned how balancing the macronutrients with the 40/30/30 plan creates a favorable hormonal response, as a result of the glucagon release triggered by the protein. Not only will this mobilize stored body fat, but the "good" eicosanoids produced will regulate the cardiovascular system.

Bio-Foods, makers of the Balance nutrition bar, sponsored two independent clinical studies, one at Pepperdine University and the other (a preliminary study as yet unpublished) at Sansum Medical Research Foundation in Santa Barbara. These studies demonstrated that the 40/30/30 formula not only improves athletic performance, aids in weight loss, and is safe for diabetes, but also raises the levels of good HDL cholesterol. The Pepperdine University double-blind, crosssover study, showed an increase in HDL of 13.5 points in just four weeks.[4]

I have lectured and written about the dangers of high-carbohydrate intake in several of my books. Fortunately the issue has also been recognized by some progressive members of the medical profession. Dr. Diana L. Schwarzbein, a Santa Barbara endocrinologist was quoted in *The Santa Barbara News* in December, 1994:

> Eating foods high in cholesterol does not increase blood cholesterol. . . . Overeating carbohydrates can lead to abnormal cholesterol levels. And foods that raise insulin levels are the ones that cause obesity, high blood pressure, high cholesterol and heart disease.

A diet high in carbohydrates is one which will put a man at risk for developing cardiovascular disease. This is especially so if that diet is made up of refined carbohydrates.

## Chromium

In the refining process, white sugar loses 93 percent of its chromium. White flour has only 23 mcg. per 100 grams of this important trace mineral, compared to the 175 mcg. per 100 grams found in whole wheat flour, if the wheat was grown in mineral-rich soil. It is well known that chromium plays an important role in sugar metabolism.

What is not so well known is that it also plays an important role in fat metabolism.

It appears that there is a link between disorders of fat metabolism and those of sugar metabolism: Practically everybody with clinical athero-sclerosis of moderate severity has a mild form of diabetes. People with moderate to severe diabetes have especially severe atherosclerosis from which most die. This association was established a number of years ago. It was discovered in 1959 that rats with reduced glucose tolerance (diabetes) were deficient in chromium. This disorder can be prevented or cured by adding chromium to the diet. It was later established con-clusively that chromium is necessary for the utilization of insulin in glucose metabolism. Subsequent animal studies indicated not only ele-vated blood sugar levels when chromium was deficient, but also ele-vated blood cholesterol levels. Both can be lowered by the addition of chromium to the diet.

When it comes to humans, chromium tends to be present in the bodies of all young people. However, according to Dr. Schroeder author of *The Trace Elements and Man* (1973), it is not detected at all in the tissues of 15-23 percent of Americans over fifty. It is present, however, in 98.5 percent of foreigners over fifty. Furthermore, **no** chromium was found in the aortas of people who died from coronary artery disease, while it was present in those who died of other causes. These findings make the inclusion of chromium in the diet vitally important for the prevention of heart disease. Chromium is found in honey, grapes, raisins, corn oil, clams, whole-grain cereals, and brewer's yeast.

In view of these findings we would be wise to limit our intake of refined foods, or better yet, to eliminate them entirely, especially white sugar and white flour. Many following the gospel of the low-fat, high-carbohydrate diet over the last decade, have overdosed on sugar.

## That Sweet Tooth

Sugar is eight times as concentrated as flour and much more deadly. The refining process has robbed it of trace minerals and many other nutrients, including the family of B vitamins. In the absence of B vitamins, carbohydrate consumption cannot take place. When carbohydrates aren't broken down properly, they ferment in the system, adding a toxic burden to the body. Sugar is, of course, a carbohydrate. And, when we consume it in its refined form, where none of the nutrients needed to metabolize it are present, the body must rob its storehouses to obtain these nutrients. As the storehouses become depleted, degenerative disease sets in.

The average American consumes over 138 pounds of sugar and high fructose corn syrup per year. That breaks down to over four dozen teaspoons daily per person! Only one-fourth of that amount is consumed at the table and for cooking. The rest is found in our foods. Not just the obvious ones like cookies, cake, candy, and ice cream, but hidden in ketchup, salad dressings, canned soups, peanut butter, luncheon meats, and canned and frozen vegetables. Even cigarettes, cigars, and pipe tobacco contain sugar! **Read labels.** There are many forms of sugar and many names for it. Avoid foods containing corn syrup and any containing ingredients that end in "ose."

As sugar consumption increases, so does heart disease. A professor of Nutrition and Dietetics at Queen Elizabeth College of London University found the following association between deaths from heart disease or heart attack (per 100,00 people) and the amount of sugar they consumed per year:

| | |
|---|---|
| 20 pounds per person | 60 deaths |
| 120 pounds per person | 300 deaths |
| 150 pounds per person | 750 deaths[5] |

Sugar raises triglyceride, cholesterol, insulin and blood pressure levels and contributes to obesity, all risk factors for the development of heart disease. It has been linked with kidney damage, premature aging, reduced immunity, migraine headaches, gallstones, tooth decay, diabetes, hypoglycemia, diabetes, birth defects, learning disabilities, and cancer. Used in the curing process, sugar adds to the addictive qualities of tobacco. Tests at Brookhaven National Laboratory found that patients on a high-sugar, low-fat diet had triglyceride levels two to five times greater than those on a low-sugar, high-fat diet.

Our liking for that sweet taste may have been nature's way of prompting us to include fruits and vegetables in our diet. Back when they were mineral rich, these foods had a sweet taste. Because of their fiber content, naturally sweet foods delay the release of sugar into the bloodstream and their minerals assist in its utilization. On the other hand, consuming sugar by itself, or any of the concentrated sugars—such as honey, barley malt, rice syrup, maple syrup, molasses—triggers an immediate insulin response and all of the attendant negative consequences.

All these sweeteners are refined products. Even "raw" sugar is only white sugar to which molasses has been added. While these foods are somewhat more nutritious than white sugar, they all raise cholesterol and triglycerides, depress immune activity, and contribute to yeast overgrowth (which can cause fatigue and a variety of mental symptoms). Excess sugar can also block the manufacture of good prostaglandins (eicosanoids) from EFAs.

### Fructose

Many people consider fructose to be a healthy alternative to refined sugar because it is a "natural" sweetener found in fruit. Over the past fifteen years, consumption of high fructose corn syrup has tripled, going from 19 pounds per person in 1980 to 56 pounds in 1994. During that same period, sugar consumption actually decreased. High fructose corn syrup is widely used by food manufacturers—in soft drinks, baked goods, jellies, jams, syrups, ketchup. Even health food stores deal in fructose—sold in its crystalline form and as an ingredient in concentrated fruit juices.

Since fructose has a low glycemic index rating, meaning that it does not convert quickly to blood sugar, nor raise insulin levels rapidly, it has been recommended by some for diabetics. However, this recommendation is invalid. The liver is the only organ that can metabolize fructose. A high-fructose diet puts a strain on the liver similar to alcohol consumption. While every cell in the body can metabolize glucose, the liver must convert fructose into glucose before it enters insulin pathways. For these reasons, fructose should be avoided by diabetics.

Another strike against fructose is that it elevates LDL (bad) cholesterol, increasing the risk of heart disease. It was found in a Department of Agriculture study conducted in 1993 that consuming as little as two to three soft drinks with high fructose corn syrup daily can elevate LDL levels.

A caveat about switching to diet sodas. Diet sodas contain aspartame (sold under the trade names of NutraSweet or Equal). Although there is no evidence linking it to cholesterol levels, aspartame has its own set of health problems. Headaches, dizziness, confusion, decreased vision, severe depression, extreme irritability, severe anxiety attacks, numbing of hands and feet, ringing in the ears, convulsions, nausea, palpitations, and marked personality changes have all been associated with ingestion of asparatame. Eighty to eighty-five percent of consumer complaints to the FDA have involved aspartame. And aspartame is not only found in diet soda. Over 1200 products, including children's vitamins, drugs, baked goods, laxatives, and chewing gum now contain aspartame.*

## WHAT THE EVIDENCE SHOWS

In terms of human evolution, sugar consumption is a new and rapidly increasing addition to our diet. In 1870, we were only consuming 11 teaspoons per person per day. Animal products were a staple part of the human diet long before heart disease escalated to epidemic proportions. If eating meat caused heart disease, we would expect to see high incidences of it in cultures that consume large amounts of meat. This has not been the case.

Among people whose native diet consists of a high percentage of animal fat are the Yemini Jews, the Eskimos, and the Masai tribesmen of Africa. All of these people enjoy good health, free of heart disease until they either migrate to Westernized cities or adopt a Western diet, heavy in sugar-laden, processed foods. Several Mediterranean societies have also been free of cardiovascular disease, despite a diet that is up to 70 percent fat.

Over thirty years ago Ancel Keys, Ph.D., discovered that people living in the southern European countries had a very low rate of heart disease. It was especially low among the people of the Greek island, Crete—90 percent lower than the U.S.—despite the fact that 40 percent of their diet was composed of fat. Olive oil, a monounsaturated fat, was their primary source of fat, with only 8 percent of the calories coming from saturated fats.

Another group of people with a very low incidence of heart disease is the Japanese from Kohama Island. These people have something in common with the Cretans: They both have a high dietary intake of linolenic acid, an Omega-3 EFA. The Cretans get their linolenic acid from walnuts and purslane (a thick-leaved "weedy" plant used in salads), while the Japanese get theirs from soybean products and rapeseed (canola) oil.

French researchers took a group of 605 patients, all of whom had had one heart attack, and placed half of them on a typical Cretan diet. They ate bread, grains, vegetables, fruit, poultry, fish, and some cheese and used only olive and canola oil for cooking. No butter or margarine was

*The Aspartame Consumer Safety Network has volumes of available information on the dangers of aspartame. They may be contacted at P.O. Box 780634, Dallas, TX 75378, (214) 352-4268.

used, but rather a spread rich in Omega-3 essential fatty acids. The other half of the patients were placed on the American Heart Association (AHA) diet, one high in polyunsaturated fats and low in cholesterol and saturated fats. Total fat was restricted to 30 percent, with saturated fat limited to 10 percent. Their progress was followed over a twenty-seven-month period, during which time the cholesterol levels, blood pressures, and weight of both groups remained about the same.

However, there was a marked difference in the number of patients having a second heart attack and surviving it:

|  | AHA Diet | Mediterranean Diet |
|---|---|---|
| Total Number of Heart Attacks | 33 | 8 |
| Number of Deaths Caused by Heart Attacks | 16 | 3[6] |

The advantages of the Mediterranean diet were so obvious that the study was prematurely ended. The patients on the AHA diet were put on the Cretan diet. By completion of the study, those on the Cretan diet showed concentrations of linolenic acid in the blood that were near to that of the natives of Crete and Kohma. The study is significant in that it demonstrates that establishing Omega-3 EFA sufficiency is more important than lowering cholesterol. It is not necessary that we adopt a Mediterranean diet (though it may be most beneficial to those of Southern European ancestry), but we do want to get plenty of Omega-3 fatty acids in our diet: Not necessarily from purslane—flax seed oil will do just fine!

## IRON OVERLOAD

The most recent heart disease culprit, iron overload, was also a new one to me. Just as I was finishing this manuscript, I got a call from my uncle, Jack Kriwitsky, who insisted I meet with him and a friend for dinner that night. At dinner, I met Jack Fox, my uncle's friend who had just returned from a conference in Florida on iron overload. He gave me a book called *The Iron Elephant* (Vida, 1992). Much of what I learned about iron is from this book. I also learned that Jack Fox had become so interested in the iron problem because of his lady friend who had the problem and discovered it quite by accident.

Plain and simple, iron can be a hidden killer that adversely affects the heart under certain circumstances. High levels of iron in the body have been linked with heart disease and hypertension, as well as with headaches, liver disorders, arthritis, diabetes, and cancer. A five-year Finnish study followed 1,900 men who had no clinical evidence of heart disease when the study began in 1984.[7] The researchers measured the amount of ferritin, a protein that binds iron in the blood. They found that for each 1 percent increase in the amount of ferritin in the blood, there was a more than 4 percent increase in heart attack risk. A ferritin level of 200 micrograms or greater more than doubled the relative risk of heart attack. Typical ferritin levels for adult males are from 100-150 micrograms. Next to smoking, the study found ferritin levels to be the strongest risk factor for heart attack. LDL levels alone were not found to be a significant risk factor, but they were significant when paired with elevated iron. Another study found iron in atherosclerotic plaques in humans. And iron promotes oxidation of LDL.

These findings underscore the importance of excluding iron supplements from the diet of men unless a need for the mineral is demonstrated through laboratory analysis. They also speak of the importance of making sure that the iron we do put into our body is bioavailable (from organic sources) so that it stays in solution and does not contribute to plaque formation. To assure this, body pH must be normalized through electrolyte balance and a balanced diet. Since meat is high in bioavailable iron, excessive consumption of it can cause a build-up of the mineral in the body, especially if pH is off balance.

Surprisingly, new research indicates that many people suffer from iron overload caused by a genetic condition known as Hereditary Hemochromatosis (HH). People with normal iron metabolism absorb no more than the amount of iron needed daily, while those with HH absorb it excessively, to toxic levels. Once absorbed, iron is not excreted. The only way iron levels can be lowered is through blood loss. Once thought to be extremely rare, HH is proving to be quite prevalent, especially among Caucasians, affecting 2 in 400.

Over a million Americans carry the gene. Roberta Crawford was one of them. It took her twenty-six years and four doctors to get a correct diagnosis. During this period of time, she was misdiagnosed, as many are, with anemia and given more iron. Her symptoms included headaches, joint pain, diarrhea, heart irregularities, and heavy menstrual bleeding. After her ordeal, Crawford formed the Iron Overload

Diseases Association* and wrote *The Iron Elephant* to help educate the public on the problems associated with iron overload.

Symptoms of excess iron can also include anemia, fatigue, low immunity, abdominal pain, lack of mental clarity, and a gray or bronze tint to the skin. Over time, the accumulation of iron in the system can cause organ damage, resulting in such conditions as arthritis, diabetes, impotence, sterility, premature menopause, cirrhosis, heart disease, and cancer.

Many people, like Crawford, are misdiagnosed, as doctors commonly make the faulty assumption that anemia is caused by low iron without doing the proper testing. Anemia can be diagnosed with a fingerprick test and hemoglobin count, but without further laboratory analysis, the cause of the anemia cannot be ascertained with certainty. While low iron levels can cause anemia, iron loading can cause it too. The most effective tests to screen for HH are those that measure serum iron (SI) concentration, the total iron-binding capacity (TIBC), and the stored iron or ferritin. Once HH is diagnosed, it is important that family members be tested, since it can be passed on genetically.

Prognosis for HH is good, especially if it is detected early before organ damage is done. For this reason, blood profiles are recommended for those men showing symptoms that may be indicative of HH.

Iron overload should be considered a major risk factor in heart disease, second only to cigarette smoking. Excess iron causes the oxidation of LDL, promoting the formation of plaque in the arteries. Becoming a frequent blood donor is the main therapy for iron overload.

## CONGESTIVE HEART FAILURE

While the death rate for heart disease has been decreasing, the number of cases of Congestive Heart Failure (CHF) have increased. According to American Heart Association statistics, the number of people hospitalized for the disease more than doubled between 1979 and 1992, going from 377,000 to 822,000. It is the most common cause of hospitalization for people over sixty-five, with 50,000 people dying from it each year and cost of care exceeding $50 billion annually.

The American Heart Association describes CHF as a condition in which the heart becomes weakened, unable to pump out all the blood

* You can contact the Iron Overload Diseases Association at 433 Westwind Drive, Dept. W, North Palm Beach, FL 33408, (407) 840-8512.

that flows through it. According to Dr. Bruce West, CHF would more appropriately be called "beriberi of the heart."[8] Beriberi is a disease caused by deficiency of B vitamins, especially $B_1$ or thiamine. Symptoms of this deficiency disease include nerve conductivity problems, weakness and muscle paralysis. Dr. West draws the parallel to CHF, describing it as a "problem of poor nerve conductivity to the heart, an almost paralyzing weakness of the heart muscle and the resultant failure of the heart muscle to be able to pump out blood."[9]

According to Dr. West, vitamin $B_4$, which has not been synthesized, nor recognized by the FDA, together with $B_1$, are vitally important for proper heart muscle function. He emphasizes the fact that all of the B vitamins are linked together with thousands of phytochemicals, plant chemicals, most of which have not been synthesized, nor even identified. Phytochemicals are needed to activate vitamins and minerals, and they are absent in isolated vitamins produced in the laboratory. We must look to whole foods as a source of supply. The alternative is to use a B complex supplement made from food and plant sources, one that is processed in such a way as to maintain the phytochemicals. The B vitamins are found in brewer's yeast, liver, and whole grain cereal. $B_1$ is also found in egg yolks, meat, fish, fowl, legumes, and nuts.

Julian Whitaker, M.D., observes that thirty years ago patients with CHF invariably had a history of heart attack that had inflicted damage upon the heart muscle. Today, however, CHF patients are presenting with no history of heart attack. Dr. Whitaker believes that the factor responsible for this and for the escalation of CHF over the last few decades is the "overuse of medications called beta blockers."[10] Beta blockers, he explains, are used to lower blood pressure. They do so by blocking the heart's ability to respond to epinephrine and adrenaline (which stimulate and elevate both blood pressure and pulse rate). These drugs lower blood pressure by weakening the heart.

Dr. Whitaker believes that, while beta blockers are useful for temporary relief of symptoms, long-term use can lead to CHF. His belief is supported by multiple references in the *Physicians Desk Reference* (a book doctors use when prescribing drugs) to possible cardiac side-effects, including heart failure from long-term use of such beta-blockers as Lopressor.

Another class of drugs commonly prescribed for high blood pressure, calcium channel blockers, is also associated with an increase in death from heart disease—a 60 percent increase. The mineral magnesium works better than these drugs as a calcium-blocking agent to prevent spasm of the coronary arteries—and it has no side effects.

Separate studies have found that supplementation with taurine, a non-essential amino acid,[11] and the mineral potassium[12] can be useful in the treatment of CHF. A deficiency of muscle potassium could not, however, be corrected if magnesium deficiency was also present.

Cardiomyopathy is a generalized term, pertaining to myocardia (heart muscle) disease. It encompasses CHF, atherosclerosis, and hypertension (high blood pressure). Cardiomyopathy can result from selenium deficiency. This was demonstrated in 1972 when "Keshan Disease," which has plagued the Keshan Province of the People's Republic of China since 1930, was found to be identical to "Mulberry Heart Disease" in pigs, known to be caused by a selenium deficiency. The soil in Keshan Province is almost totally lacking in selenium.

One of the many functions of selenium in the human body is the protection of the cellular membranes of both skeletal and cardiac muscle fibers from free radical damage. A selenium deficiency is intensified by exercise and by a high intake of polyunsaturated fats. This important trace mineral is added to commercial food for pets, laboratory and farm animals, but not to food meant for human consumption. The pigs may not be getting Mulberry Heart Disease anymore, but we are!

## HYPERTENSION

Hypertension is an abnormal elevation of blood pressure that can lead to heart and kidney diseases or stroke. It affects one out of four men. Actual physical ailments such as kidney infection, obstruction of a kidney artery, adrenal disorder, or constriction of the aorta account for about 10 percent of the cases. These conditions can usually be corrected. For the majority of people, however, the exact cause of hypertenison is not known. The condition is then referred to as "essential hypertension." A major factor associated with hypertension is atherosclerosis, which obstructs the flow of blood through arteries. Stress is also an important factor, for it causes contraction of arterial walls.

When blood pressure is high, the body is out of balance. Drugs used to lower pressure won't correct the basic imbalance (electrolyte imbalance) and indeed can further disturb it. Side effects of hypertension drugs can include cardiac problems. Diuretics are the most commonly prescribed medication for hypertension. And they are the safest. But you should be aware that diuretics can rob the body of minerals essential to heart function. As Dr. Earl Mindell explains in his *Joy of Health* newsletter (April 1995, p.3):

> Most diuretics lower blood pressure by preventing the
> kidneys from returning sodium to the blood, which
> increases the volume of urine. The result is to reduce
> the volume of fluid in the blood and in other cells of
> the body. Unfortunately, as the urine carries sodium
> out of the body, it takes other minerals salts with it,
> most importantly potassium and magnesium—two
> minerals that are essential to your heart health.

Since one of the purposes of taking diuretics is to reduce sodium levels,
a sodium-restricted diet is recommended for hypertensives. Sodium
intake can be reduced just by avoiding packaged and processed foods.
There's no need to avoid foods such as celery that are naturally high in
sodium—in fact, it has been found that there's a substance in celery that
can relax the walls of blood vessels. Regular table salt, which is highly
processed and devoid of trace minerals, should be eliminated entirely.
It can be replaced with a totally unrefined, mineral-rich salt such as
Celtic Sea salt* and used in moderation. This type of salt will not cause
fluid retention. Most sea salts found in health food stores are processed
to some degree and should be avoided.

Salt restriction will not lower blood pressure if potassium levels are
low, which, of course, it most often is with people who take diuretics. Symptoms of potassium deficiency include muscle cramps, irregular heartbeat, constipation, insomnia, weakness, and nervous disorders. The level of this important mineral can be increased by eating
such potassium-rich foods as fruits, vegetables, whole grains, lean
meats, legumes, and sunflower seeds. Drinking fresh fruit and vegetable juices is an excellent way to get plenty of potassium. Those on
diuretics should take in around 2,000 mg. of potassium daily from
food sources.

Diuretics not only cause potassium loss, but also excretion of other
minerals such as calcium and magnesium. Inadequate levels of calcium,
magnesium, and potassium can cause contraction of blood vessels,
resulting in elevation of blood pressure—which puts us right back
where we started! To replace these minerals, I recommend regular use
of a good multi-mineral formula in conjunction with the Trace-Lyte
electrolyte formula. (See Appendix C for specific products and pro-

* Celtic Sea salt is available through the Grain and Salt Society. Call (916) 872-5800.

gram). Long-term diuretic use can result in impaired glucose tolerance due to the loss of potassium and chromium if these important minerals aren't replaced.

Spending more time outside in the sun can help to increase vitamin D levels. This, together with increased intake of potassium and calcium will cause the body to excrete more sodium. Vitamin C and bioflavonoids can help maintain or restore the health of blood vessels strained by the increased pressure they're under.

Weight loss can favorably influence blood pressure. In fact, for every 2 pounds of weight lost, blood pressure should drop 1 point in both systolic (top number) and diastolic (bottom number) readings. Most people with hypertension are overweight, weighing an average of 29 pounds more than people with normal blood pressure. Even 5 pounds of excess body weight can contribute to high blood pressure. Weight loss can be achieved without dieting, simply by following the 40/30/30 eating plan.

Regular exercise is also helpful in reducing blood pressure: Those who exercise are 34 percent less likely to develop hypertension than those who don't. Strenuous exercise is not necessary. Dr. Mindell tells us that "just a brisk half-hour walk 3 to 4 times a week can lower blood pressure by 3 to 15 points in just 3 months."[13]

Hypertension, like diabetes, is associated with insulin. Both conditions can be caused by insulin resistance. In insulin resistance, the pancreas (even in the diabetic) produces plenty of insulin, even too much. That insulin just isn't getting to the cells because it is blocked by fat. In addition to avoiding the "bad" fats (trans fats, refined oils, too much unsaturated fat) and replacing them with EFAs, insulin resistence can be prevented or corrected by reducing carbohydrates which trigger the insulin response.

In his *Health and Healing* newsletter of December 1994, Julius Whitaker, M.D., tells us that a trace element, vanadium, inhibits the synthesis of cholesterol and that this mineral, in the form of vanadyl sulfate, given in large doses, can eliminate diabetes and certain forms of high blood pressure, apparently by making cells more responsive to insulin. The intriguing thing is that improvement is sustained even after supplementation is discontinued.

Apart from the traditional risk factors associated with hypertension— excess weight, stress, lack of exercise, smoking, and poor diet—we can add "exposure to environmental toxins" such as cadmium to our list of risk factors.

## TOXIC TO THE HEART

Our environment—the air we breathe, the food we eat, the water we drink—is increasingly tainted with contaminants. Among them are a class of toxic minerals known as heavy metals which include lead, cadmium, aluminum, and mercury. None of these metals belong in our bodies (except for a minute amount of aluminum), but have found their way there through our polluted food, air, and water supplies.

Among other disorders, heavy metals have been linked with heart disease. Lead toxicity is associated with cardiovascular dysfunction, arteriosclerosis, and atherosclerosis; aluminum toxicity can paralyze the heart; mercury, even in small amounts, can damage the heart, as well as other organs; and cadmium toxicity gives rise to hypertension. Cadmium replaces zinc in the arterial walls, leading to reduced flexibility and strength in the arteries. A build-up in arterial plaque results, as the body coats the arteries in an effort to prevent formation of aneurysms.

## TWO VITAMIN-LIKE COMPOUNDS THAT HELP THE HEART

**Carnitine:** A vitamin-like substance once considered to be a non-essential amino acid. The body can synthesize carnitine from the essential amino acids lysine and methionine. The conversion cannot take place, however, without adequate iron and vitamin C. Higher levels of carnitine are found in the blood of men than women, suggesting that men have a higher need for it.

Carnitine may be obtained from the diet in the form of muscle and organ meats, dairy products, and legumes. It is not present in vegetable protein, however, and vegetarians may be deficient due to low levels of the precursor, lysine, in the diet.

Carnitine stimulates fat metabolism, regulates triglyceride levels, increases HDL, and decreases LDL. It can be of potential value in a number of heart disorders. By normalizing carnitine levels through supplementation, the heart is assisted in better utilizing its limited oxygen supply.

It has recently been demonstrated that carnitine can also help protect cells from free radical damage, though it is not actually an antioxidant: Rather than neutralizing free radicals, it helps cells recover from the damage they inflict.

Coenzyme Q10 (CoQ10): Like carnitine, CoQ10 is another vitamin-like compound that can be synthesized in the body. It is a substance found in all of the cells of the body, with greatest concentration in the liver and the heart. Tissue levels decrease with age. CoQ10 plays a major role in energy production in the body and a deficiency of it can cause or aggravate many conditions, including heart disease, diabetes, and periodontal disease.

The heart may be particularly vulnerable to CoQ10 deficiency because it is one of the most metabolically active tissues of the body. A CoQ10 deficiency has been demonstrated in up to 75 percent of myocardial biopsies in patients with various heart diseases. Conditions such as angina (heart pain), mitral valve prolapse, high blood pressure, and CHF can benefit from CoQ10 supplementation. A University of Texas study using CoQ10 with CHF patients found that 78 percent improved and their survival rate was higher than those receiving standard treatment.

CoQ10 can lower triglycerides and total cholesterol, while raising HDL. It appears to be useful as a weight-loss aid due to its ability to stimulate the mitochondria and increase the fat-burning process.

The best food sources of CoQ10 are meat, some fish and vegetable oil. Other good sources include rice bran, wheat germ, soy and other beans.

## MAGNESIUM: THE HEART MINERAL

Every single male that I work with is directed to take extra magnesium. I firmly believe that magnesium is the key to many of our current maladies, including heart disease.

Magnesium is the second most common mineral in our cells. It plays a major role in protecting the heart. Deficiency of this important mineral has been linked to hypertension, arrhythmias, and CHF. Insufficient magnesium can cause coronary artery spasms that will reduce blood and oxygen flow to the heart and result in a heart attack. It has been found that individuals who have died suddenly from heart attacks have had very low levels of magnesium in their hearts. Death from ischemic heart disease (caused by obstruction of arteries) is more common in areas where soil and water have low levels of magnesium. It has also been shown that magnesium is needed for the body to use insulin properly.

A recent Gallup survey found that 72 percent of adult Americans fail to meet the Recommended Daily Allowance for magnesium. RDA for adult males is 350 mg. per day. The survey also showed that magnesium consumption decreases with age. Low levels of magnesium not only increase the risk of developing high blood pressure and heart disease, but also increase susceptibility to insomnia, muscle cramps, diabetes, kidney stones, and cancer.

Compounding the problem of low magnesium intake is the high calcium intake of Americans. Magnesium should optimally be taken in equal proportion to calcium. Americans have been urged to eat more dairy products as a source of calcium, and we're doing so, much to our detriment. Dairy products contain nine times as much calcium as magnesium.

Early man adapted to an environment rich in magnesium, but lacking in calcium by developing mechanisms for storing the latter. We still store calcium more efficiently than magnesium so we don't need as much of it in our diet as we've been led to believe. What little magnesium we do consume in the SAD is further depleted by a diet high in sugar and alcohol, which increases magnesium excretion through the urine.

Magnesium is abundant in whole foods—tofu, legumes, nuts, seeds, whole grains, leafy greens, and, sea vegetables—but is lacking in refined foods, eaten so abundantly in the SAD. We can get ample calcium in our diets without including dairy products that are not well absorbed due both to their low magnesium content and their high phosphorus content.

## OTHER HEART-SMART NUTRIENTS

Since the oxidation of LDL is proving to be an important contributing factor in heart disease, the antioxidant nutrients become an important weapon against the disease. Flavonoids, found in fruits and vegetables are powerful antioxidants. A five-year study involving 500 men in the Netherlands found that those who consumed the most flavonoid-rich foods were half as likely to have a heart attack or die from coronary disease as those eating the least amount of flavonoids.

One study on vitamin E involved 39,910 healthy men. It began in 1986 and lasted four years. During that period of time, 667 of the men developed coronary artery disease. The study found that those men who had the highest level of vitamin E intake had 40 percent less risk of coronary disease compared with those men with the lowest intakes. Risk reduction was seen only for men taking in at least 100 IU per day, and the use of supplements for at least two years seemed to be necessary to achieve this protection.

Another study interviewed patients following angioplasty (a procedure that dilates blocked coronary arteries) and found that those who regularly took vitamin E experienced restenosis (reoccurrence of blood vessel narrowing) at a rate of only 15.8 percent compared to a rate of 30.7 percent in those not taking the vitamin.

Antioxidant enzymes—such as Superoxide dismutase (SOD) and Glutathione peroxidase—scavenge free radicals 7-10 times faster than antioxidant vitamins and minerals. Supplemental antioxidant enzymes, however, have low bioavailability and can be quite costly. Good food sources of the antioxidant enzymes are wheat sprouts, alfalfa, barley, wheat grass juice, and bee pollen.

A true electrolyte formula, which includes trace minerals in a crystalloid form, will also enhance this ability. Trace minerals are needed for the production of the SOD factors: Manganese and zinc stimulate the production of SOD. Glutathione peroxidase is also mineral-dependent: It requires selenium. Both Glutathione peroxidase and SOD are normally present in large amounts in heart tissue to protect it from oxidative damage.

Selenium deficiency can reduce the antioxidant defenses of the heart. It is the mineral activator of the vitamin E complex. Selenium and vitamin E work together to protect the heart and a deficiency of either can be damaging, but a deficiency of both is observed to produce more severe oxidative damage.

Another extremely potent antioxidant is pycnogenol. Rather than being a specific nutrient, pycnogenol is actually a group of substances—proanthocyanidins—found in a particular type of flavonoid or bioflavonoid. It has been found to scavenge free radicals 50 percent more effectively than vitamin E and 20 percent more effectively than vitamin C. Proanthocyanidins greatly increase vitamin C activity, strengthening collagen in the blood vessels and increasing capillary resiliency. This, in turn, improves circulation.

It was found by Dr. David White at the University of Nottingham in England that the proanthocyanidins prevent the oxidation of LDL. While vitamin E scavenges free radicals only in fatty areas of the body and vitamin C scavenges them only in watery areas, pycnogenol scavenges them in both. It also has anti-inflammatory activity.

Pycnogenol comes from pine tree bark and grape seed. Studies show that it is completely non-toxic and highly bio-available.

I've already mentioned some of the B vitamin family members that play an important role in protecting the heart—$B_1$, $B_4$, and choline, which is necessary for fat metabolism. The body's fat metabolism can also be impaired by a severe deficiency of biotin. Such a deficiency is rare, but can be brought on by eating large amounts of raw egg white.

Another B vitamin, niacin ($B_3$), has been used for many years to treat high cholesterol and elevated triglycerides. High doses of niacin can cause not only flushing, itching, and an upset stomach, but also increased blood glucose, uric acid, and liver enzyme levels. For this reason, one should be under the care of a health care professional when using large doses of this vitamin. It should not be used by people with a history of gout, liver dysfunction, or diabetes.

We've heard from the aspirin people that an aspirin a day will keep clotting away. And while there have been studies showing that aspirin can be helpful in preventing clotting that can lead to heart attacks, aspirin can have serious side-effects, such as bleeding of the stomach lining when taken regularly. New studies link aspirin to macular degeneration, the number one cause of blindness in people over fifty-five. A safe, natural alternative to aspirin for achieving anti-blood clotting results is bromelain, an extract from pineapple. Bromelain breaks down arteriosclerotic plaques and relieves angina pectoris through enzymatic action. Fourteen patients with angina were given 400-1000 mg. daily of bromelain and all were asymptomatic within ninety days, some in as few as four days, depending on severity. Systemic enzyme therapy can also be used to improve blood fluidity and circulation.

Antioxidants and flavonoids help to improve circulation, strengthen blood vessels, and decrease clotting, thereby lowering the risk of atherosclerosis, heart disease, and stroke. Certain herbs contain these compounds. Most notable of them is hawthorn, a member of the rose family. Anthocyanidins and proanthocyanidins are part of the flavonoid content of hawthorn giving the plant antioxidant properties. Hawthorn decreases cholesterol, inhibits atherosclerotic plaque build-up, lowers blood pressure, and dilates coronary vessels, which improves blood flow and increases blood supply to the heart muscle. This herb has been shown to increase the force of the heart's contraction and prevent arrythmias. It works well with many heart medications, but should not be used with beta blockers.

Another herb that has been demonstrated to decrease cholesterol and triglyceride levels is garlic. These findings have been the result of studies on animals and humans conducted for over thirty years. Consuming 600 mg. per day (half of a clove) of garlic powder for two weeks reduced significantly the susceptibility of fats in the blood to oxidation. Garlic has powerful antioxidant properties and can lower cholesterol by at least 10 percent in less than one month. It also has the ability to prevent blood from clotting. Be aware, however, that raw garlic can lower blood sugar.

Cayenne can play an important role in supporting heart function. It has been used traditionally by herbalists as a crisis herb, in coronary and other emergencies. The herb is also useful to take on a regular basis (a quarter teaspoon taken three times daily) to stimulate the circulation and prevent heart attacks and stroke. It will also help prevent headaches, indigestion, colds, flu, and arthritis. Both cayenne and garlic have been used to lower blood pressure in hypertension.

## PUTTING IT ALL TOGETHER

Heart disease is a product of modern "civilized" society, where stressful lifestyles and diets of devitalized foods create the conditions for its development. As with all of the illnesses discussed so far, changes in your dietary habits are essential for improving the health of your heart.

High dietary cholesterol does not correlate with an increase in heart disease. Increased sugar consumption does. So you need to switch your focus from all those "No Cholesterol" labels and start looking for all the sugars that are hidden in foods from Rice-A-Roni to Jiff peanut butter.

The way to a man's heart is through his stomach certainly holds true in more the its original intention. The healthy way to protect your heart are not only your food, but monitoring risk factors like your cholesterol ratio, weight, controlling stress, magnesium and EFA deficiencies, and iron overload. There's a lot that you can control here. Your health is in your hands.

Please refer to Appendix C for specific guidelines on a supplement program that puts together findings and recommendations from this chapter.

# CHAPTER 7

# SUPER NUTRITION
# FOR SUPER SEX

You can be a sexual dynamo at any age. All you have to do is generate some excess energy—that is, energy in excess of that which is required to maintain the vital functions of the body. Sexual energy is surplus energy. It can be abundant in the healthy male, regardless of age. Health is intimately linked with lifestyle and diet, and **you** are in control of these factors. You have the power to enhance your vitality and your sexuality. All you need is the right information on how nutritional and environmental factors affect sexual functioning. I will discuss effective ways to deal with decreased sex drive, impotence, premature ejaculation and infertility.

Nutritional deficiencies can leave you feeling fatigued, listless and depressed, with little, if any, energy left for sexual activity. Our bodies were not designed to handle **chronic** stress. While we can handle acute episodes of stress and recover, the increased stresses that today's man is under in our fast-paced, competitive society leave many continually exhausted. Nutritional needs skyrocket during stressful periods. When these needs go unmet, additional stress is placed upon the body. As the nutritional gap widens, energy and stamina diminish. When we talk about restoring or enhancing sexual functioning, we're really talking about bringing energy and vitality back into the body, which is what getting healthy is all about.

## THE HEALING POWER OF SEX

There is a definite correlation between good health and good sex. When we're healthy, we're in balance. Balance confers on us, among other things, vigor and vitality, as well as a properly functioning hormonal system. The result is normal, healthy functioning.

Not only is good health necessary for proper sexual functioning, it would appear that the reverse is also true: A fulfilling sex life enhances physical, as well as emotional health. According to Alexander Lowen, M.D., executive director of the International Institute for Bioenergetic Analysis in New York City, both men and women who are sexually satisfied, are much less likely to develop heart disease. Studies support this. One, involving 131 men, ages 31-86 who had been hospitalized for heart attack, found that two-thirds reported suffering from sexual difficulties just prior to their heart attacks.

Sex is therapeutic for us. It helps relieve stress. By doing so, it may also enhance the body's immune function. The stress response involves a reduction in T-cell count and beta endorphin levels. Our T-cells are immune cells that fight off invading germs or other foreign bodies. Endorphins are brain chemicals that help us tune out pain. They're produced in large numbers during strenuous exercise and during sex. When stress is reduced, endorphin and T-cell production increase. Therefore, by alleviating stress, sexual activity can enhance immunity and reduce pain. The increased endorphin production that results from sexual activity may explain why it tends to relieve back pain and arthritis. In addition to blocking pain, endorphins also produce feelings of euphoria and exhilaration.

## IMPOTENCE

An estimated 30 million American men suffer from impotence. Impotence literally means "no strength." It is a condition of erectile failure, where the male is either unable to get an adequate erection or unable to sustain it long enough to successfully complete intercourse. The penis has "no strength."

According to J. Douglas Trapp, M.D., a board certified urologist and consultant to the Osborn Foundation Impotence Resource Center in Augusta, GA, about 15 percent of males everywhere are impotent. He claims that successful treatment is available for over 90 percent of the men so affected. Nonetheless, 60 percent of impotent men put off going to the doctor for at least a year.

A large advertisement run in a small town newspaper by a clinic specializing in treating impotency, states that impotence is the "most common medical disorder in the world—almost as common as the cold, but much more treatable." It goes on to say that 95 percent of their patients are treated with medication. What it **doesn't** say is that a very large number of drugs can **cause** impotence. Among them are several classes of medication for hypertension, ulcers, antihistamines, seizure medications, medication for nausea, sedatives, antidepressants, and tranquilizers. Abuse of street drugs, alcohol, and smoking can also be major causes of physical impotency.

It has been found that 90 percent of men with impotence are or have been heavy cigarette smokers (another good reason to quit!). A study reported in 1994 in the *Journal of Epidemiology* involving 4,462 Viet Nam veterans found that current smokers had 50 percent more reported impotence than non-smokers. These percentages are significant.

Before 1980, the prevailing medical opinion about impotence had been that it was caused largely by psychological problems. Today, however, the tides have turned, and most cases of impotence are now believed to stem from organic disorders. If a man is able to get an erection during sleep or masturbation or with a different partner, organic causes can be ruled out and emotional causes should be assessed. The primary causes of psychological impotence are depression, marital problems, job stress, and performance anxiety. Immaturity and low self-esteem can also be contributing factors.

In addition to prescription and street drugs, alcohol, and smoking, impotency can be caused by the following physical factors:

Circulatory insufficiency
Disorders of the nerves (such as MS, paralysis from an accident)
Hormonal deficiency
Surgery
Radiation for pelvic cancer
Severe kidney failure
Severe chronic diseases (such as cancer, cirrhosis of the liver)
Cadmium toxicity
Intense exercise

This last factor, intense exercise, was found in a Michigan Medical Center study to lead to a drop in production of hormones involved in potency, fertility, and sex drive.

## CIRCULATORY INSUFFICIENCY

Of the above factors, circulatory insufficiency is the most common cause of impotence in American men. Arteriosclerotic plaque on the walls of penile arteries can result in diminished blood supply to that organ. A study following the progress of 3,250 men, ages 26 to 83 found that high total cholesterol and low HDL tend to correlate with erectile dysfunction.[1] So keeping your arteries clear of plaque is not only good for your heart, it's good for your sexual performance as well.

Because of their ability to stimulate vascular flow to the penis, yohimbe and ginkgo biloba are two herbs that are often used to treat impotence. Ginkgo biloba extract was given to a group of men who had been unresponsive to traditional drug therapy. In a six-month period, half of the group regained potency. One 40 mg. capsule taken daily can produce results in two months, though it may take up to six months to regain full potency.

I have many clients who absolutely swear by yohimbe. Its active ingredient, yohimbine, is derived from the African yohimbe tree. Yohimbine dilates surface blood vessels and stimulates the release of norepinephrine, which opens the vascular door to the penis. Yohimbine also decreases the latency period between ejaculations and has been demonstrated to increase libido. In a study done at Stanford University, three groups of rats (normal, virginal, and impotent) were injected with yohimbine. Afterwards, nearly half of the sexually inactive rats began copulating, while copulation in the normal group nearly doubled.

The usual dose of yohimbe bark standardized extract is 50 mg., one or two capsules daily. Yohimbine can increase heart rate and cause a slight increase in blood pressure, creating a feeling of nervousness, but is without serious side effects. Dr. Christian Barnard, pioneer in heart-transplant surgery, reports that three out of four heart transplant patients had immediate return of sexual potency after taking yohimbine.

George, a fifty-four-year-old architect, reluctantly came to see me at his wife's insistence. Six months previous, he had undergone bypass surgery. After his convalescence, he was having a difficult time in the bedroom. He's been following a moderate exercise program and really watching his diet. George had a notorious sweet tooth, but since his bypass, he had been careful with both sugar and bad fats.

I started him on the Super Nutrition Sex Formula that included yohimbe bark standardized extract as well as other sexually supportive ingredients. I recommended one a day to start, and suggested he might want to take an additional one before an amorous evening. By the end of one week, his wife called to tell me the new vitamins I was giving him were beginning to work.

The B vitamin niacin can also improve blood flow to the penis. It is one of several nutrients that has a "chelating" effect. Chelation is a process that occurs naturally in the body. Certain nutrients bind with material obstructing the arteries and escort it out of the body. Other natural chelators include vitamins $B_6$ and C, the minerals magnesium, manganese, and selenium, DMG (discussed later in this chapter), the enzyme bromelain, and the mineral salts orotic acid and aspartic acid.

The material that clogs arteries is made up largely of mineral deposits, laid down when minerals go out of solution. This happens as a consequence of pH imbalance. Since pH is regulated by electrolytes (including their trace mineral factors), they too can be viewed as chelating agents. In fact they are superior chelating agents. By correcting pH, they correct the basic conditions that give rise to the problem. Garlic, onions, and high-fiber foods also assist in the natural chelation process.

## HORMONAL DISORDERS

When one thinks of hormones in relation to impotence, testosterone is probably the first to come to mind. Actually, the pancreas, thyroid, and adrenal glands all produce hormones that effect human sexual functioning and response. In fact, diabetes causes 90 percent of hormonal impotence, and the hormone involved here is, of course, insulin.

The adrenal glands, which produce the sex hormones, working together with the thyroid produce and maintain the body's energy levels. And extra energy is what you're after for peak sexual performance. Our bodies were not designed to handle chronic stress, the kind of stress many men live with today. When the body experiences stress, it goes into an alarm reaction. The adrenal glands begin to hyperfunction. Once the stress is removed, the adrenals quiet down and return to their normal function. This is what the body was designed to do.

But when stress continues the adrenal glands draw energy from the body's reserves. Nutrients not supplied by the diet will be siphoned off from reserve areas. When stress becomes a way of life, the body simply becomes exhausted. Reserves of energy and nutrition are totally depleted. Those who live with constant, unending worries about finances, family, health problems, divorce, etc. use up excessive amounts of nutritional reserves every day. And chances are if you're stressed out, you aren't eating right to begin with.

Stress to our physical bodies comes in many different forms. In addition to the emotional and mental stress we commonly think of, physical stress, including any physical injury, illness, overwork, or lack of sleep affects the adrenals. Any chemical substance, whether from environmental pollutants or diets high in refined and overprocessed foods, must be detoxified by our bodies and this too puts stress on the adrenal glands. Job stress, lack of or excessive exercise, use of stimulants such as coffee, sugar, and "recreational" drugs all contribute to burn-out.

And when the adrenals "burn out," passion's flames are extinguished. If you're tired when you get up and spend the better part of your day spiking you tired adrenal glands with caffeine, nicotine, sugar, sodas, or excessive exercise just to get through another day, there's not much energy left to spike you into sexual action in the evening.

Underproduction of thyroid hormones, hypothyroidism, as mentioned in Chapter 8, leads to many health disorders, among them fatigue and impotence. Again, the lack of energy necessary for peak sexual performance and enjoyment is missing in a man suffering from hypothyroidism.

Testosterone deficiency interferes with erections and suppress sexual desire. Testosterone levels decline with age. As they decline, so does sexual desire and performance, especially in men. It is testosterone that determines sex drive—in women, as well as men. At age twenty-five, the average free testosterone level in men is about 200 pg/ml. At age eighty, it's only about 10 pg/ml. While testosterone levels decrease with age, the incidence of impotence increases as men get older. The following statistics show percentage of impotence for each decade of life between ages forty and eighty:

age 40    2 percent
age 50    5 percent
age 60    18 percent
age 70    27 percent
age 80    75 percent

As you might discern from these figures, there is a male menopause. Called andropause, its onset is more subtle than that of menopause in women, but it can, nonetheless, be difficult because of the symptoms it can produce. In addition to impotence, these include weakness, stiffness, pain, nervous exhaustion, loss of muscle tone, irritability, and profuse sweating, with intolerance to heat. According to William Campbell Douglass, M.D., "many of these problems will completely disappear with proper testosterone therapy."[2] "Proper" means correct doses (small) and correct form (avoid methyl-testosterone, as it harms the liver). The doses of testosterone used to counteract the symptoms of andropause are much smaller than those used by athletes who take steroids to increase muscle mass. In such large doses, testosterone can actually destroy the sex drive.*

One way to confirm the onset of andropause is by measuring levels of a hormone called Follicle-Stimulating Hormone (FSH). It is a pituitary hormone that controls sex hormone secretion in both men and women. Andropause is heralded in by an increase in FSH levels, which can be measured in blood or urine collected over a twenty-four-hour period. Another way to verify onset of andropause is through the "estrogen urine test." Here the amount of male estrogen production is reflected in a day's output of urine. Amounts in excess of 20 mcg. indicate that the change has taken place.

## COMBATTING IMPOTENCE WITH NUTRITION

Super nutrition plays a big-time role in increasing performance and your ability to handle stress. While good nutrition won't solve your marital problems or take away on-the-job pressures, it can increase your ability to handle the stress. Nutrition is probably your strongest ally when it comes to maximizing your manhood.

---

* For information on balanced hormonal therapy contact Broda O. Barnes Research Foundation, P.O. Box 98, Trumbill, CT 06611, 203-261-2101.

On the old high-carbo diet, the brain isn't getting its fair share of its only fuel, glucose. The glucose in the body is being used as an energy source to run the rest of the body. The result is the development of hypoglycemic symptoms, many of which are emotional in nature. These can include fatigue, insomnia, headaches, nervous habits, and mental disturbances. Adopting the 40/30/30 eating plan and using unprocessed whole foods will have a stabilizing effect on blood sugar, mood swings, attention span, focus, and long-term energy.

An intake of the right kinds of EFAs will help the body produce tissue-like hormones called prostaglandins (a form of eicosanoid) that regulate sexual response. The gonads "make use of fatty acids for hormone production and for the transfer of neurogenital impulse waves to the brain."[3] Insufficient prostaglandins, due to lack of the Omega-6 EFA (GLA), can produce such sexual dysfunctions as insufficient ejaculate and infertility. Vitamin $B_6$ helps convert linoleic acid into prostaglandins. Evening primrose oil and borage are excellent sources of GLA. They provide specific fatty acids that produce heightened sexual response. Spirulina is also rich in GLA, as well as being an excellent source of complete and highly digestible protein. It has been used to treat impotency, lack of libido, and premature ejaculation.

For optimal sexual functioning, the thyroid and adrenal glands, as well as testicular function must be supported nutritionally. Vitamin E and zinc nourish the sex glands, while adrenal support is provided by vitamins A, C, E, B complex (especially $B_2$ and pantothenic acid), and the EFAs. The thyroid gland is supported by iodine and the B vitamins (especially $B_1$ and pantothenic acid).

Remember: The proper balance of macronutrients produces "good" eicosanoids that regulate the cardiovascular system, and circulatory insufficiency is the most common cause of impotence in our culture. American men can therefore both protect their hearts and enhance their sexuality by adopting a balanced eating plan. Adding an abundance of fatty fish to the diet may also help, as studies have shown that they increase blood levels of EPA and DHA (two Omega-3 EFAs). This may, in turn, help prevent cardiovascular problems and enhance sexual activity.

## VITAMINS AND MINERALS

**Selenium:** Nearly half of the selenium in a man's body can be found in his testicles and in portions of the seminal ducts alongside the prostate gland. Since selenium is scarce in our food supply and vital to proper sexual functioning, men need to make sure that they get plenty of this important trace mineral in their diet. Foods high in selenium include butter, herring, tuna, wheat germ and bran, Brazil nuts, brewer's yeast, whole grains, and sesame seeds.

**Manganese:** This essential trace mineral is commonly deficient in impotent men, as revealed in hair analysis. Nuts, seeds, and whole grain cereals are rich in manganese.

**Zinc:** Vital to the production of testosterone, a deficiency can result in impotence, as well as reduced sperm count. Zinc also helps to guard against cadmium toxicity which can lead to impotence. Cadmium toxicity is common in smokers. A man's ability to absorb zinc declines with age, and the mineral is destroyed by drugs, alcohol, coffee, and smoking, as well as by infections. Good food sources include pumpkin and sunflower seeds, seafood (especially oysters), organ meats, brewer's yeast, soybeans, mushrooms, herring, eggs, wheat germ, and meats.

**Vitamin E:** Dubbed the "sex vitamin," vitamin E works with selenium as an antioxidant. When the penis is erect, it is engorged with blood that carries vital oxygen. Vitamin E assists in the transport of that oxygen and prevents its oxidation. Good food sources of this antioxidant vitamin include peanuts, almonds, cold-pressed oils, eggs, wheat germ, organ meats, desiccated liver, sweet potatoes, and leafy vegetables.

**Vitamin C:** Vital to the sex glands, particularly as a man ages. If an insufficient amount is obtained from the diet, the sex glands will steal it from other body tissues. If there is none to steal, sex drive will diminish or vanish, as sex-gland functioning drops or stops. Foods rich in vitamin C include citrus fruit, rose hips, acerola cherries, sprouted alfalfa seeds, cantaloupe, strawberries, broccoli, tomatoes, green pepper.

**Vitamin A:** Helps maintain testicular tissue. It is found in liver, eggs, yellow fruits and vegetables, fish liver oil, and dairy products.

**The B Complex Vitamins:** The B vitamins influence the production of testosterone. $B_1$ and $B_2$ help support the thyroid and adrenal glands respectively. Pantothenic acid is needed for both of these glands that produce 98 percent of the body's energy. When they're underactive, fatigue and diminished sex drive can result. Folic acid works in conjunction with testosterone to develop mature sperm. Para-aminobenzoic acid (PABA) has been successfully used in treatment of Peyronie's Disease, a condition characterized by extreme curvature of the penis, which makes erection quite painful. The best food sources for the B complex vitamins are brewer's yeast, liver, and whole grain cereals.

**Phosphorus:** The first mineral to be recognized as directly involved with sex drive, phosphorus is found in curries, chutneys, and hot sauces, all of which provide stimulation (in the form of irritation) to the sex organs. Truffles, underground fungi, purported to have aphrodisiac effects, contain phosphorus. It is present in lecithin in the form of phospholipids (a combination of nitrogen, fatty acids, and glycerol) that help promote the secretion of sex and other hormones. Lecithin can be produced in the body only in the presence of the B vitamins, especially $B_6$. Brewer's yeast, wheat bran and germ, pumpkin, squash, and sunflower seeds are all very high in phosphorus.

## OTHER NUTRIENTS

**Tyrosine:** People with low levels of the brain chemicals norepinephrine and adrenalin are prone to depression and loss of libido. The amino acid, tyrosine, is directly involved in the production of these chemicals that control mood, sex drive, and energy level. Tyrosine is also a precursor to the neurotransmitter, dopamine, that is so intimately involved with sexual drive.

There is evidence that small doses of tyrosine are more effective in increasing brain levels of neurotransmitters than large doses. Doses of 1,000 mg. morning and night can be administered when blood levels are low, with a gradual increase to 2,000 mg. twice a day. This amino acid has also been shown to lower blood pressure and depress appetite. Supplemental tyrosine is not recommended for anyone with melanoma, nor for individuals taking MAO-inhibiting drugs. (It should also be avoided by pregnant women).

**Aloe Vera Juice:** Due to the properties of its principle oils, vitamins, minerals, amino acids, and other ingredients aloe vera juice is said to have sexually stimulating properties. It's also very healing for internal organs. One half cup of the clear gel, taken daily is recommended for this purpose.

In the "Birds and the Bees" equation, the bees seem to be far more important. They produce three products that can benefit men sexually. Pollen contains natural hormonal substances that stimulate and nourish the reproductive system and help increase sexual stamina. Royal Jelly can be of benefit for impotence, as well as sterility. And honey, too, increases potency, as well as the body's production of sex hormones. Go easy with such concentrated sweet substances, however, for they can create havoc with blood sugar levels by triggering the insulin response.

**Dimethylglycine (DMG):** An over-the-counter food compound, once known as pangamic acid or vitamin $B_{15}$, DMG is a "non-fuel nutrient" that "acts as a cofactor, aiding vitamins, fats, hormones and proteins in completing their metabolic action or cycle."[4] DMG aids in detoxification of the body by increasing oxygen utilization at the cellular level. This results in increased muscle tone of the organs, including the sexual organs. It restores elasticity and strength to the penis.

DMG also helps combat fatigue at doses of one or two 90 mg. tablets daily. It improves circulation and normalizes blood levels of several hormones by stimulating the adrenal glands, important to sexual functioning. Additionally, DMG increases cellular production of lecithin (found in high amounts in male reproductive fluid), which helps promote sex hormone secretion.

## HERBS

Herbs seem to work best if taken in cycles, rather than on a continuous basis. This way the body remains more responsive to their effects. You may wish to rotate and alternate herbs and herbal combinations for optimal effectiveness.

**Ginseng:** By helping it overcome stress and fatigue, recover from deficiencies, and regain strength, ginseng benefits the entire body. It does this, in part, by supporting the adrenal glands. Ginseng comes in many varieties—Korean, Chinese, Siberian, and American. The Manchurian variety (from China) is particularly rejuvenating to the male reproductive system, as it stimulates the endocrine glands to increase testosterone production.

The herb has been studied extensively. Laboratory tests with mice and rats showed that following injection with a ginseng extract, the animals copulated more frequently. Increased growth of organs, especially the gonads, was also noted. As a stimulant, it may produce side-effects such as insomnia, irritability, and nervousness, especially if taken over a long period of time.

**Saw Palmetto:** Described in Chapter 5, saw palmetto can also be useful in treating impotence. It not only helps to build strength, but is considered by some to be an aphrodisiac.

**True Unicorn Root:** Reported to be an excellent herbal medicine for impotence, unicorn root has also been used to promote fertility in both sexes.

**Sarsaparilla:** An herb rich in phytosterols (plant steroids), sarsaparilla also nourishes sex hormones and therefore can be of use in treating impotence.

Bayberry, black cohosh, and goldenseal can help support thyroid function. So can sea vegetables because of their high-mineral content. Lack of iodine and the amino acid phenylalanine (which breaks down into tyrosine) can cause a lack of thyroid hormones. Zinc, manganese, and the B vitamins are also needed for the gland to function properly.

Other herbs, besides ginseng, that support the adrenal glands include licorice root, hops, passionflower, and skullcap. Stress exhausts these glands and depletes the body of vital minerals including calcium, magnesium, zinc, potassium, sodium, and copper. Eating sea vegetables such as dulse, hijiki, arame, and nori, is an excellent way to replace these minerals and improve the health of the adrenals. The B vitamins, as mentioned, and vitamin C also support adrenal function.

## MECHANICAL DEVICES, INJECTIONS, AND IMPLANTS

For those men who require assistance with erectile function due to a mechanical defect in the penis, there are numerous devices on the market that can assist. These devices mechanically produce an erection. One is a condom device that produces the erection through a simple suction action. There are also vacuum devices available. In these a suction tube is placed over the penis to draw blood into it, then a rubber constriction ring is applied, trapping the blood inside. The erection produced in this manner is somewhat wobbly, but will be sufficient to permit intercourse.

An alternative to these devices is penile injection. Here a smooth muscle relaxant is self-injected into the base of the penis, causing it to engorge with blood. Depending upon the combination of drugs used and the dose, the erection can last from half hour an hour to an hour and a half. Some men report quite satisfying results with this procedure. Others find the method an unacceptable option.

A final alternative lies in surgical implants, where a rod is inserted into the penis. There are three different designs, ranging from semirigid to completely inflatable. In one model, inflation and deflation is achieved by squeezing the scrotum. Implants have been in use since the '70s. Increasingly good results are claimed by the medical profession, notwithstanding the wave of litigation seen a few years ago, resulting from improperly placed or defective devices.

Treatment of impotence is a growing medical specialty. Those clinics offering it generally employ the above three procedures, implants, injection, and mechanical devices, as well as hormone therapy and vascular bypass surgery. Of these treatment options, hormone therapy may sound like the most acceptable; however, if the cause of the problem is vascular, rather than hormonal, it would be of little benefit. While hormone therapy may be a more "natural" approach than the others, bear in mind that hormonal output is largely determined by nutrient input. Balancing macronutrients, EFAs, and electrolytes can do much to restore hormonal balance in the body, possibly obviating the need for exogenous hormones.

Not counting the cost of diagnostic work-up, the price of treatment in a medical clinic specializing in impotency can range from $500 per year for medication to more than $25,000 for surgery requiring a hospital stay. Impressive "cure" rates of 90-95 percent sometimes claimed often refer to injection therapies that many men decline. Impotency clinics don't generally offer less costly, less invasive nutritional therapies as described in this chapter. Such approaches come closer to offering a "cure," if we construe the word to mean "correction of the underlying problem," rather than symptomatic relief.

## PREMATURE EJACULATION

It has been found that physical disorders are rarely the cause of premature ejaculation. In order to determine if an ejaculation is premature or timely, we need some guideline as to how much time it normally takes for a man to ejaculate. It might surprise you to learn that,
in the average sexual encounter, only three minutes elapse from the
man's first thought of having sex until the act culminates in ejaculation. For a woman, the average time between arousal and orgasm is
thirteen minutes.

Doctors have sometimes prescribed circumcision for premature ejaculation because it decreases sensitivity in the penis. A majority of men
in our society are already circumcised, however. It may be helpful for
men to wear a condom—or two or three—during intercourse to avoid
overstimulation that may lead to premature ejaculation. Some men
choose to masturbate earlier in the evening before having intercourse.
The reasoning here is that the first erection does not last as long as subsequent ones that will have more staying power.

It can also be helpful for men to learn to control the sensations that
lead up to ejaculation. One technique for this is to practice delaying
ejaculation during extended foreplay. The partner squeezes the penis
lightly when the man reports an approaching sensation of orgasm. An
alternative is the "stop-start" technique that substitutes interrupted
foreplay for squeezing when the male senses that ejaculation is forth-
coming.

Some cases of premature ejaculation can be caused by high histamine
levels. Elevated histamine is associated with allergies. Men with allergies therefore may tend to ejaculate sooner than men without them.
Calcium and the amino acid methionine can be used to help lower
blood histamine.

## INFERTILITY

It may be normal for fertility to decline with age. Sperm production
normally decreases by more than half from ages twenty to eighty. But,
infertility is not normal and is a sign of a depleted system. Infertility
affects approximately 15 percent of all couples. Those unable to conceive generally want to be tested to get to the root of the problem.
They are usually advised to wait at least at a year before doing so, as

conception occurs among 80 percent of fertile couples after one year of trying. One-third of infertility is a result of female sterility, one-third results from male sterility and the other one-third stems from conditions of both partners. Although men are no more often the source of the conception problem than women, it is recommended that they be tested first, as procedures involved with their testing are simpler. Understand, however, that infertility screening is costly and often unproductive. Medicine is able to find the sources of infertility in only 60 percent of the men tested.

Before embarking upon screening, couples may want to apply some nutritional wisdom. Correcting lifestyle habits such as smoking and drinking, modifying stress, and taking nutritional supplements can help protect genetic material in the sperm and ova. Couples unable to conceive may also want to follow the advice of medical experts: Have intercourse every other night from day 10 to day 18 of the menstrual cycle, avoid the use of lubricants and the practice of douching afterwards.

The average man today produces only half as much sperm as his grandfather did. A study conducted in 1992 found that sperm counts among men in industrialized nations declined 50 percent in a fifty-year period. These findings are consistent with more recent studies published in the *New England Journal of Medicine* and the *British Medical Journal*. They report a decline in sperm count between 33 and 41 percent in recent years.

Male infertility can be caused by congenital defects (absence of spermatic duct, undescended testes), hormonal imbalance, drugs (street and prescription), chemicals, radiation, infections, the existence of sperm antibodies, varicocele (a varicose vein draining a testis), and retrograde ejaculation (a common result of prostate surgery).

It would appear that a major cause of decreased sperm production among men virtually everywhere in the "civilized" world is the widespread use of industrial and agricultural chemicals, such as Dioxin. They are chemically similar to estrogen and have a toxic effect upon the body by acting in an estogen-like manner. When pregnant women are exposed to these hormone-mimicking chemicals, their male offspring are born with fewer sperm-producing Sertoli cells. Increasing numbers of reproductive-tract abnormalities have resulted from exposure to these chemicals in our food, air, and water.

Hey, and watch those tight jeans. There may be a connection between tight jeans and restricted circulation to the family jewels that leads to reduced sperm counts.

Even when sperm count is normal, reduced motility (swimming ability) can contribute to infertility. Where both are present—low sperm count and lowered motility—a man's chances of being infertile are greatly increased. Both motility and fertility of sperm are proportionate to the amount of vitamin E in the semen. Experiments on rats have shown that when a group was fed a diet adequate in all other respects, but lacking in vitamin E, the first generation of rats became partially sterile, the second generation completely sterile. Vitamin E is an important antioxidant nutrient that is largely lacking in processed foods. I recommend supplementation with 400-600 I.U. daily in the form of mixed tocopherols. Selenium, as the mineral activator of the vitamin E complex, is also needed—300 mcg. per day recommended.

Vitamin A is also important to fertility. It promotes the formation of a higher number of sperm in the ejaculate. Vitamins C, E, and the B vitamin folic acid as well as the EFAs are all important to sperm production.

Vitamin $B_{12}$ has also been successfully used in treating male sterility. It, plus the B vitamin inositol, as well as vitamin C and the minerals calcium, magnesium, zinc, and sulfur are all found in healthy sperm and so may be necessary for fertility.

Another nutrient that benefits both sperm count and motility is carnitine. In a recent study[5] three grams of carnitine were given daily to 100 infertile men with sperm motility problems. At the end of four months, increased sperm motility and count were noted, with the most dramatic improvements occurring in those men who entered the study with the poorest sperm motility.

The essential amino acid arginine can also be useful in doses up to eight grams. Four grams per day increases sperm count in 80 percent of men with low counts. It is not suggested in doses over 30 mg., however, for men with a history of schizophrenia, for it can aggravate symptoms through its chemical action. Arginine is also contraindicated in cases of herpes simplex infection. Men with such infections should also avoid arginine-rich foods, primarily nuts and seeds, and may want to consider supplementing their diet with lysine.

Studies have shown that if more than 20 percent of sperm are clumped together (sperm "agglutination"), conception will not take place. In one study, men given 500 mg. of vitamin C every 12 hours showed an 11 percent decrease in sperm agglutination after three weeks. Vitamin C guards against sperm damage that can cause birth defects and childhood illnesses.

As well as creating problems for the heart, iron overload can cause infertility, as well as impotence. Men suffering from these conditions may want to rule out Hereditary Hemochromatosis through the laboratory tests mentioned in Chapter 6.

While hot tubs and saunas are often used for relaxation and to enhance sexual encounters, you should know that they can lead to reduced sperm counts.

Histamine is a chemical in our cells and blood that controls ejaculation. B vitamins, especially niacin and folic acid, as well as fatty acids, can help in some cases of infertility, for they raise blood histamine levels. Men too low in histamine can't achieve ejaculation. Inversely, men with high levels of histamine, may ejaculate prematurely.

## ENHANCING THE ENCOUNTER

Aphrodisiacs, named after Aphrodite, the Greek Goddess of love, beauty and fruitfulness, are substances that increase sexual arousal. Down through the ages, about 2000 substances have been purported to have aphrodisiac effects. Dr. Morton Walker tells us that "the physiological basis for some aphrodisiacal claims is that when the substance is eaten, drunk or rubbed on the body, it acts on nerve centers in the brain to decrease inhibitions."[6] Any of the foods or other substances mentioned in the preceding pages as useful in restoring libido can be considered as aphrodisiacs.

According to the teachings of Oriental medicine, the kidneys govern sexual vitality. They can be irritated by excessive intake of coffee, alcohol, fatty foods, or emotional stress. The kidneys—and therefore sexual energy—are nourished by warmth. Eating too many cold foods such as fruits and salads or drinking iced beverages, especially in cold weather can "cool one's passion."

To warm the kidneys and nourish sexual energy, one needs foods like beans; whole grains; green, leafy vegetables; and seeds. Seeds not only contain the germ of life, but are an excellent source of zinc, found in abundance in seminal fluid. Oysters, also rich in zinc, are said to have been the "love tonic" of Casanova. Eggs—organic, "fertile" eggs—have also been considered to have aphrodisiac properties, as has garlic, artichokes, mushrooms, and caviar. Fish have been long thought to stimulate sexual activity and, for that reason, priests were at one time forbidden to eat them.

Many of the culinary spices, because of their warming and gentle, stimulating nature are considered to be aphrodisiacs. These include ginger, cloves, cardamom, anise, caraway, nutmeg, vanilla, and cinnamon.

Aphrodisiacs can also include substances applied externally to the genitals. Medicine has employed the use of nitroglycerine paste applied directly to the penis to help impotence. It does not have this effect taken orally, however.

Musk oil, from the musk ox, has traces of sheep testosterone in it. Ambergris is a gray, waxy substance excreted in the intestines of sperm whales. Either of these oils may be rubbed into the penis (after washing and drying it) one hour prior to intercourse to enhance the experience. These oils "cause a contractile reaction in the muscles of the penis, so erectile tissues can remain stiff."[7] They can also be applied to the clitoris.

Musk and ambergris also have a pleasant scent. Women react most to musk-like smells. Men and women both can become sexually stimulated through the olfactory sense, it seems, in subconscious reaction to chemicals called "pheromones." Most animals and humans secrete these chemicals as a component of perspiration. About 10 percent of men secrete a pheromone called androsterone in their perspiration. It has been proven that women find these men exceptionally appealing, being aroused subconsciously by the pheromones they sense.

Actually, women secrete androsterone too. It is produced in the adrenal glands of both sexes. It's also found in the vaginal labia and in the foreskin of the penis. Women's reaction to the pheromone is most pronounced, for they're a thousand times more sensitive to smells than men are.

In the '70s, an aerosol spray containing androsterone came to the U.S. from Great Britain under the name "Bodywise." Theoretically, such a product could help correct sexual dysfunction.

The sense of smell can be further stimulated by the use of essential oils in erotic encounters. The aphrodisiac oils include jasmine, ylang-ylang, cinnamon, aniseed, clove buds, ginger root, nutmeg, peppermint, pepper, and rose. A few drops of these oils can be placed onto the mattress.

To further enhance the atmosphere, orange, magenta, and purple decor are said to increase arousal. Candle light, soft music, and flowers can help, too.

During orgasm, both men and women experience a "sexual flush." It is the result of histamine release in the body. The B vitamin, niacin, produces a similar flush. It also increases sexual lubrication, by stimulating activity in the mucus membranes of the mouth and vagina. Taking 50-150 mg. of niacin fifteen to thirty minutes prior to a sexual encounter can enhance the sexual flush and mucus membrane activity.

## SUMMING IT UP

See Appendix D for a supplemental program for impotence. Important points to consider when planning a program for super sex:

Good overall health is vital to proper sexual functioning. Both are influenced by physical and psychological factors.

Adrenal and thyroid support are vital to restoring sexual energy.

Most impotence is caused by organic problems, chief of which is circulatory insufficiency. Yohimbe and ginkgo biloba are herbs that can improve blood supply to the penis. Chelating nutrients can also help: $B_6$, vitamin C, magnesium, manganese, selenium, DMG, bromelain, orotic acid, aspartic acid. Electrolytes are essential.

Sperm counts have declined dramatically over the last fifty years due largely to the widespread use of industrial and agricultural chemicals.

Important fertility nutrients include vitamin E, selenium, vitamin A, vitamin B complex (especially folic acid, $B_{12}$, and niacin), EFAs, arginine, carnitine, vitamin C, calcium, magnesium, sulphur, inositol, and zinc. These last five are found in healthy sperm. It is important to rule out iron overload as a cause of both sterility and impotence.

# CHAPTER 8

# SUPER NUTRITION
# FOR HAIR LOSS

By now you know that Super Nutrition can make a big difference in many areas of your life. Can it make you leaner? Yes. Can it improve your sex life? Yes. Can it improve your athletic performance? Yes. Can it stop hair loss? Again, the answer is yes. You can keep a full head of hair provided you take the right steps early on. And, even if thinning has set in, there's a lot you can do to minimize further loss. Research is shedding new light on the causes of hair loss in men. Consequently, effective new treatments are being developed. Armed with a nutritional arsenal, you will be able to prevent or reverse hair loss.

An estimated 30 million men experience loss or thinning of their hair as they age. About the same number are affected by impotence. Though the two are not related, what they have in common is that hormonal factors feature heavily in their cause. I'll look at these factors, as well as other causes of hair loss in men in the pages that follow. Some nutritional, medical, and other approaches to correction of hair loss problems will also be explored.

## NORMAL HAIR LOSS

Hairs fall out and are replaced by new ones on a regular basis. Loss of 50-100 hairs per day is normal. Problems result when these lost hairs either aren't replaced right away, aren't replaced at all, or are replaced with inferior quality hair.

There are three phases of hair growth known as anagen, catagen, and telogen. The anagen phase is the growing phase. It normally lasts two to six years. The catagen phase is a transitional one. It should last only about three weeks. Hairs that have entered the telogen, or resting phase, remain dormant in the scalp for two to four months, at the end of which time the old hair is pushed out by a new one growing in the same root. In men with hair loss problems, however, the telogen phase is extended, lasting for several years or for the remainder of their lives.

In the form of hair loss known as Male Pattern Baldness (alopecia hereditaria), normal (terminal) hairs are replaced by nearly invisible, fine, light hairs (vellus). Over the years, more and more terminal hairs are replaced by these barely visible vellus hairs, as the hair root decreases in size. A man with such thinning hair may appear to be bald, but this is not the case. In true baldness, the roots of the hair have withered, hair follicles died.

## MALE PATTERN BALDNESS

Male Pattern Baldness (MPB) comprises 90 percent of hair loss cases. It affects approximately half of all males in Western industrialized countries. MPB is "androgenetic" hair loss, meaning that it has to do with genes and male hormones. It is believed to be caused by a "baldness gene" that is passed on by one parent. DHT is also thought to be a primary factor in shrinking of hair follicles and subsequent hair loss. DHT, you'll recall, is dihydrotestosterone, a metabolite of testosterone, which increases with age and has been associated with prostate problems. That hormones are somehow involved with hair loss in males is certain, for eunuches never lose their hair. Castration, then, is a sure form of prevention, albeit an extreme one!

MPB first shows up as a receding hair line that can manifest at a very early age, sometimes shortly after a man has reached sexual maturity. The pattern in MPB is for hair loss to be confined to the top of the head. Why it is limited to this area is not known. It has been found that balding men are deficient in an enzyme known as aromatase. When this enzyme is present in sufficient quantity, follicles grow hair. When there's not enough aromatase, follicles switch off.

## OTHER TYPES AND CAUSES

Alopecia hereditaria or androgenic alopecia (MPB) is just one of about three dozen different types of alopecia, all characterized by partial or total hair loss. Alopecia universalis is loss of hair all over the body. Alopecia areata is a sudden loss of hair in patches on the head, beard, and other parts of the body. Among the possible causes of these different types of hair loss are:

| | |
|---|---|
| poor circulation | radiation |
| acute illness | skin disease |
| high fever | sudden weight loss |
| trauma | iron deficiency |
| diabetes | thyroid disease |
| excessive vitamin A intake | vitamin deficiency |
| poor diet | heavy metal toxicity |
| tight connective tissue in scalp | drugs |
| parasites | stress |

Drugs that can cause hair loss include chemotherapeutic agents, antibiotics (penicillin, sulfonamides, mycin), heparin (an anticoagulant), and carbimazole (a hyperthyroid drug).

While poor circulation may contribute to hair loss, it alone does not appear to be a necessary and sufficient condition to cause the problem. If it were, then stroke victims would lose their hair, hair transplants wouldn't work and bald men wouldn't bleed profusely when cut on the scalp. Nonetheless, activities aimed at improving circulation, such as massage, exercise, and the use of a slant board (fifteen minutes per day) can be useful adjunctive therapies when paired with other corrective measures.

One of the newest and most innovative approaches to stimulating hair growth involves the use of electrical stimulation. In a Canadian study, thirty men received low-powered pulses of electrical stimulation emitted from a device resembling a hooded hair dryer. Such treatment, given twice a week for twelve minutes, resulted in the growth of new hair or prevented hair loss in twenty-nine of the subjects. Re-growth of hair occurred in 96.7 percent of the group with **no future loss**. Such treatment may help to loosen connective tissue that can cause hair follicle strangulation.

## THE ROLE OF NUTRITION

Vitamin deficiencies that can lead to hair loss include insufficient inositol and PABA. These B vitamins protect hair follicles. When animals are put on a diet lacking inositol, their hair falls out. When it's added, the hair grows back. Hair loss for male animals is twice that for females, indicating a higher need among males. PABA not only protects hair follicles, it has also been found effective in restoring natural hair color. When deprived of this vitamin, the hair of laboratory animals turns gray. Prematurely graying hair can also be caused by a deficiency of the amino acid phenylalanine, which is enzymatically related to melanin, the hair color pigment. Biotin, folic acid, and pantothenic acid can be helpful in restoring hair color. Also, when animals lack biotin in their diet, hair loss results.

All of the B vitamins are important to the health and growth of the hair. A high potency B complex tablet (100 mg.) taken three times daily, with extra amounts of biotin, pantothenic acid, $B_6$, niacin, and inositol is recommended. $B_6$ deficiency will cause hair loss. Niacin will stimulate circulation. Pantothenic acid will help offset the effects of stress, as it supports adrenal function.

Although iron deficiency can be a cause of hair loss, men should not take supplemental iron unless an iron deficiency is firmly established through laboratory testing (as described in Chapter 6) because of the dangers of iron overload. Recommended amount of iron is 15 mg. Liquid iron tonics seem to be the best absorbed and are not constipating.

Vitamin C (3-8 grams daily) can aid in improving scalp circulation, as can DMG (90 mg. three times daily), and CoQ10. CoQ10 (60 mg., three times daily) will also increase tissue oxygenation. Vitamin E (400-1200 I.U. daily) is another nutrient that will improve circulation to the scalp through increased oxygen uptake. Zinc (15-50 mg.) and raw thymus glandular can stimulate hair growth by enhancing immune function.

Large doses of vitamin A (100,000 I.U. or more) taken over a long period of time can result in hair loss; however when the vitamin is discontinued, the hair loss stops. Vitamin A treatments (especially Accutane) can also cause hair loss.

All of the amino acids, as constituents of protein, are needed for healthy hair. Hair is 95-98 percent protein, as are nails. The sulfur-containing amino acids, cysteine, and methionine, are of particular importance. The former is involved in maintenance of hair strength. Cysteine supports liver function and promotes keratin formation. The preferred form of cysteine is N-Acetyl Cysteine. Try 500 mg. twice daily. Sheep given 1 gram per day of cysteine increased their wool production by 14 percent. Methionine (500 mg. twice daily) can help prevent hair from falling out. While adequate protein is essential to healthy hair, excess protein can lead to mineral depletion that may cause hair loss.

EFAs from flax seed oil and evening primrose oil are essential to the health of the hair. Deficiency can cause it to become extremely dry and thin and insufficient EFAs can result in hair loss. I recommend using one to two tablespoons per day of flax seed oil with about 50 mg. of $B_6$ to assure absorption plus anywhere from four to six capsules of evening primrose oil (500 mg.).

For your hair's sake, it is also vitally important to supply your body with nutrients that will support the thyroid gland. If the thyroid is underactive—and almost 40 percent of Americans are walking around with underactive thyroids—this can lead to hair loss. Hypothyroidism is a major factor in hair loss and should not be overlooked.

## HYPOTHYROIDISM

Hypothyroidism, underproduction of hormones of the thyroid gland, is characterized by the following symptoms:

| | |
|---|---|
| fatigue | dry, scaly skin |
| sensitivity to cold | dull, dry hair |
| loss of appetite | constipation |
| slurred speech | impotence |
| numbness, tingling in extremities | low sperm count |
| hair loss | recurrent infections |
| myxedema (dropping, swollen eyes) | night blindness |
| impaired intellectual capacity | |

Hypothyroidism can be the underlying cause of many reoccurring illnesses. In the elderly, the condition is often mistaken for senility. Hypothyroidism may be hereditary, or it may result from an iodine deficiency, or it may be connected to silver/mercury dental amalgams, according to Hal Huggins, D.D.S.

Many men today (and women too) have underactive thyroid glands. Iodine is an element with a very high "specific gravity." The higher the specific gravity of an element, the stronger the gastric juices must be in order to **extract** and **assimilate** the element. The strength of gastric juice is reflected in pH, which in turn is regulated by electrolytes. Lacking the trace minerals needed for electrolyte formation, pH balance is upset and therefore gastric secretions are not strong enough to utilize iodine, even when it is amply supplied in the diet. Therefore, electrolytes, as well as iodine are vitally important to proper thyroid function. Sea vegetables are good for your hair and your thyroid. Kelp and dulse are both excellent sources of organic iodine, and all sea vegetables are rich sources of other trace minerals that help keep your electrolytes sparking.

A simple way to test yourself for an underactive thyroid gland is to take your armpit temperature first thing in the morning. This method was developed by Broda Barnes, M.D., a heart specialist and endocrinologist. Place a shake-down-type thermometer next to your bed before retiring. Upon awakening, before rising, place it under the arm and lie still for fifteen minutes. A reading under 97.6 degrees F. may be indicative of hypothyroidism. Repeat the procedure several mornings and take an average of the readings. If it is 97 degrees or less you may want to consider taking a raw thyroid glandular. Armour thyroid is recommended, though available only upon prescription.

The amino acids, tyrosine and phenylalanine, can be useful in treating hypothyroidism. Tyrosine is a precursor of thyroid hormones. It is derived from phenylalanine, which also gives rise to dopamine, norepinephrine, and epinephrine. Take 500 mg. capsules of phenylalanine (up to three daily) or tyrosine (four to ten capsules daily in two or three equal doses) on an empty stomach.

Also extremely important for proper thyroid function are all of the B vitamins. There are over a dozen in the naturally occurring complex and not all have been synthesized. Therefore, in addition to taking a B complex supplement, I recommend adding foods that are rich in these vitamins to the diet. Whole grains are a good source. Brewer's yeast is excellent. The family of B vitamins improves cellular oxygenation and energy.

It is imperative that the man with hypothyroidism avoid fluoride and chlorine, as these block iodine receptors in the thyroid gland. Drinking water purified by reverse osmosis or distillation will remove fluoride and chlorine. When using RO or distilled water, remember to replenish the minerals using a liquid electrolyte formula (Trace-Lyte).

The following foods should be eaten in moderation and always cooked:

| | |
|---|---|
| soybeans | cauliflower |
| peanuts | kale |
| cabbage | Brussels sprouts |
| broccoli | watercress |
| rutabaga | turnips |

The above foods contain goitrogen, a chemical that blocks iodine absorption by the thyroid gland. The reason that these foods should always be cooked is that cooking inactivates goitrogen. The diet must also contain adequate protein, for lack of protein can inhibit thyroid activity.

Be aware that sulfa drugs and antihistamines can depress thyroid function and so should be used only under a doctor's order.

## PARASITES

Parasites are not a well recognized cause of hair loss. Medical texts list diarrhea and malabsorption as symptoms of parasitic infection. Progressive, contemporary researchers are finding that parasites can produce a wider array of symptoms that can also include:

| | |
|---|---|
| constipation | digestive complaints |
| overall fatigue | muscle cramps |
| irritability/nervousness | disturbed sleep |
| joint pain | allergies |
| persistent skin problems | post-nasal drip |
| teeth grinding | Irritable Bowel Syndrome |
| anemia | gas, bloating |

Any degenerative disease can be associated with parasites. They create a mucus overlay in the gut that blocks absorption, so that we're unable to fully utilize the nutrients we take in. Parasites can contribute to hair loss because of their immunosuppressive effect. Any man experiencing hair loss who also has one or more of the above symptoms and has ruled out other causes of hair loss may want to investigate the possibility of parasitic infection.

Many Americans hold the erroneous notion that parasites can only be a problem for those who travel to exotic places. Parasites are, in fact, a here-and-now problem. This fact was brought home in a research paper that appeared in June 1994 in *The American Journal of Tropical Medicine and Hygiene*. The paper summarized findings from a study conducted by the Center for Disease Control and Prevention in Atlanta, which showed that both in 1987 and again in 1991, stool examinations by state diagnostic laboratories revealed parasites in 20 percent of all samples.

Among the most common of the microscopic organisms found in the study were Giardia lamblia, Entamoeba coli, and Entamoeba histolytica. Since these parasites were identified using standard stool analysis techniques, we may assume that the actual incidence of parasitic infection is even greater than the study suggests, for there is a 60 percent chance of missing parasites even when three consecutive standard stool analyses are performed. It takes specialized testing techniques to reduce the number of false negative results. Even then, there is still a good chance of error. Parasites tend to hide in the lumen (lining) of the intestines and aren't easy to coax out. They live in other organs and in the blood, as well.

Parasites started making the headlines in the '90s in connection with the Desert Storm veterans. Then in 1993 they again came to our attention when the microscopic organism, Crytosporidium, found its way into the city water supply in Milwaukee, WI. Four hundred thousand people developed stomach ailments and diarrhea, and 104 died. The following year, the presence of the little critter in New York City's water supply was documented on NBC's television show, "Dateline."

According to the EPA, Cryptosporidium is currently the leading cause of waterborne illness in the U.S., appearing in 80 percent of our surface water and 28 percent of drinking water samples. It poses a serious threat, especially to those with immunosuppressive disorders. Their exposure to just a few of these organisms can cause death. Another prevalent water borne parasite is Giardia lamblia. Neither it, nor Cryptosporidium, are killed by chlorination. However, in November 1994, the EPA required all urban water systems to test for both of these parasites.

Parasites can be brought to our shores by international travelers and immigrants. They can spread through restaurants where immigrants are frequently employed in food preparation and day care centers where workers contact contaminated feces. Some parasites are sexually transmitted, some are passed on to us by our pets, others are carried by "vectors," such as mosquitos.

The problem of parasitic infection is much more widespread than we've suspected. Most physicians don't expect to find parasites and therefore don't look for them. Even if they did, they're hard to find. The problem, therefore tends to be underdiagnosed—also misdiagnosed, since parasite symptoms tend to mimic other diseases. If the problem is correctly diagnosed, it is often treated with drugs (such as Flagyl, Vermox, Iodiquinol, and Atabrine). These can cause such side effects as nausea, mental disturbances, and liver problems.

Alternative treatments make use of such parasite fighting herbs as garlic, pink root, black walnut, butternut, Ficus, mugwort, and wormwood for the larger parasites. The smaller ones can be eliminated with grapefruit seed extract and enzymes like protease, papain, and bromelain, which break through their mucus overlay. These herbs may be taken alone or in combination with herbal laxatives such as senna or cascara sagrada. Generally capsules or tinctures are taken three times a day for about two weeks, with a rest period of about five days. The cycle is then repeated once or twice more, depending upon symptoms.

The key to keeping parasite-free is building a strong immune system. We can't do this without sufficient hydrochloric acid in the stomach. HCl production tends to decline with age and with a vegetarian diet. Also, men with type A blood are more genetically prone to achlorhydria, a condition where the stomach does not produce enough hydrochloric acid. Anywhere from two to four capsules or tablets of HCl with meals can help correct the problem.

Staying away from sugar, even fruit sugar, and especially refined sugar, is very important, for parasites are drawn to it as much as we are. Perhaps the most important thing we can do to eliminate or prevent parasites is to keep a clean colon that is well populated with beneficial bacteria. Eating fiber-rich fruits, vegetables, and whole grains and taking lactobacillus supplements can help us in this regard. It is also important to minimize the ingestion of substances that will destroy friendly bacteria. These include antibiotics, caffeine, fluoride, chlorine, mercury (as found in silver dental fillings), and refined carbohydrates.

Parasites are one of many factors that can contribute to hair loss by suppressing immunity. To rule out parasitic involvement, you'll want to find a doctor who uses a lab that does either the purged stool analysis or the mucosal swab test, as these are more reliable than the standard stool analysis.*

## STANDARD TREATMENT

Up until relatively recently, the only suggestion that dermatologists had to offer to remedy hair loss was to avoid stress, get plenty of rest, use medicated shampoo, and maybe take vitamins (usually a totally inadequate multiple). That all changed in 1989 when Upjohn Co. received approval to market their minoxidil lotion, Rogaine. Minoxidil was not originally formulated to stimulate hair growth. It was used for hypertension and was widely prescribed by cardiologists.

According to Michael Oppenheim, M.D., "around 1980, a number of formerly balding cardiologists became remarkably hairy."[1] New hair growth was, however, apparently not limited to the head, but sprung up on the forehead, ears, and other places where hair is not supposed to grow. **And**, hair growth was not the only side-effect of minoxidil. In tablet form, the blood pressure medicine can cause salt and water retention, angina, rapid heart beat, and inflammation of the sac that surrounds the heart.

While it is unlikely that these symptoms would occur in men from use of the lotion, Rogaine, there is some possibility, especially for men with heart disease. Rogaine could also have adverse effects when used in conjunction with blood pressure medications. According to the *PDR Family Guide to Prescription Drugs* the following additional side-effects may occur from Rogaine:

| | |
|---|---|
| aches and pains | bronchitis |
| dizziness | facial swelling |
| arthritis symptoms | changes in blood pressure |
| changes in pulse rate | flaking scalp |
| fluid retention | anxiety |
| chest pain | ear infections |
| genital infections/irritation | back pain |
| blood disorders | depression |
| eczema | growth of excess body hair |

*If you have trouble locating a parasite specialist, you can call Uni-Key Health Systems at 1-800-888-4353 to order a state-of-the-art parasite test kit that has been made available to my readers and clients through an association between my office, Uni-Key, and a certified parasite laboratory. You can perform the test at home and the results can be quite helpful for detecting this difficult-to-diagnose condition.

| | |
|---|---|
| bone fractures | diarrhea |
| exhaustion | headache |
| hives | nausea |
| increased hair loss | conjunctivitis |
| pounding heartbeat | lightheadedness |
| redness of skin | vision changes |
| runny nose | vomiting |
| sexual dysfunction | weight gain |
| skin irritation/other allergic reactions | |

Scalp irritations and cardiovascular disease will increase the absorption of Rogaine, as well as increasing the chance of side-effects. Systemic side-effects can result from using too much of the lotion.

Minoxidil lotion is designed to be rubbed onto the scalp. It stimulates new hair growth by blocking the action of testosterone on hair follicles, reversing their shrinkage. However, if they have shrunk too much, minoxidil won't work. For this reason, Dr. Oppenheim believes that the drug is best used as a preventative. He recommends that men start using it at age eighteen and take it **for the rest of their lives!** Twice a day applications produce noticeable results in six months unless the man is totally bald, in which case it may not work at all. The more hair on the scalp, the more will be generated as a result of using the lotion.

The standard formulation of minoxidil is a 2 percent solution. Dr. Oppenheim advises that this formulation be used for one year. If results are not satisfactory at the end of that time, he recommends obtaining a special prescription for a 5 percent solution.

So, medicine's pet "cure" for baldness involves using a powerful drug every day of your life, and upping the dose if it doesn't do the job. When we consider the cost (about $100 per month) and the overwhelming number of possible side-effects of using minoxidil on an ongoing basis, plus the nutrient depletion resulting from the use of drugs, there is certainly ample reason to look for a natural alternative. Understand that although minoxidil is rubbed into the skin, rather than ingested, it still gets into the bloodstream very efficiently. The fact that it is applied topically makes it no less toxic. Any drug that must be used indefinitely is obviously not correcting the cause of the problem and so cannot properly be called a cure.

Hair transplants represent an optional way to replace lost hair. This is actually a surgical procedure that can be quite costly and painful.

There is also the risk of infection and the disadvantage of living with
unsightly scabbing wounds until they heal over. Even the successful
hair transplant often looks unnatural, and results can therefore be dis-
appointing. And, once again, nothing has been done to correct the
cause of the problem.

## ALTERNATIVE TREATMENTS

In addition to the electrical stimulation treatments mentioned earlier,
I'll discuss two other alternative hair loss treatments that have been
researched extensively and shown to be efficacious.

First, we have a topical product called Thymu-Skin.* As the name
implies, a central ingredient is thymus extract, purified calf thymus
extract. Other immune-enhancing ingredients are included in the formula, along with a number of botanicals, such as aloe vera, nettle, and
birch. Vitamins A, B, and F (fatty acids) are also present.

The product is applied to the scalp twice a day, like minoxidil. Unlike
minoxidil, however, its usage tapers off with time. Twice-a-day applications are recommended for four weeks, after which time they can be
reduced to once daily for six to eighteen months, depending upon
severity of hair loss. Thereafter, the product can be used every other
day and then reduced to twice a week as results dictate. The application
of the lotion should be accompanied by a brisk two to three minute
massage and hair should be washed twice weekly with Thymu-Skin
shampoo.

Studies on Thymu-Skin have been conducted by Dr. med. Thomas
Rabe, professor in the Dept. of Gynecology and Endocrinology at the
University of Heidelberg, Germany, by professor Dr. med. M.
Hagedorn at the University of Darmstadt in Germany and at least a
half dozen other notable physicians at reputable clinics in Germany
and Vienna. Several of these have been oncology (cancer) clinics where
it has been established that no hair loss will result from mild or moderate chemotherapy if Thymu-Skin is applied one week prior to, as
well as during, treatment.

The exact mode of action of the product is unknown, but it is
thought that the increased immunity resulting from absorption of the
thymus extract through the skin of the scalp stimulates follicles to produce tiny new hairs that will eventually grow into terminal hairs. As

* Available through Yarel Biological 1-800-257-5602.

with most other treatments, Thymu-Skin will not produce new hair growth on those areas of the scalp where hair follicles have died. As long as roots are still intact, hair loss can be stopped and hair growth reactivated. This has been proven in "thousands of patients," according to professor Dr. med. M. Hagedorn who claims that "clinical studies on patients who were losing hair caused by alopecia androgentica (pattern baldness) showed that Thymu-Skin treatment was successful in 95 percent of the women and 67 percent of the men. Therapeutic success ratios increase with longer periods of treatment."[2]

Another product that has been successfully used in stimulating hair growth is called simply "The Formula."* It evolved out of research conducted at the University of Helsinki Medical Hospital in Finland. Researchers noted that shaved laboratory mice to which they had applied a polysorbate-type solution grew hair at a faster rate than those mice to whom no solution was applied. This observation gave birth to a six-year-research project on hair growth that culminated in the development of "The Formula."

The product utilized a three-step approach to stimulate hair growth. The first step is the "cleansing" phase in which the hair follicle is cleansed of DHT, sebum, and other clogging secretions. The second step is the "washing" phase in which an all-natural shampoo is used. This shampoo includes polysorbate-type ingredients and can be used daily without weakening the hair. Finally, in the "activating" phase, a supplement-like activating solution containing twenty-two amino acids is used two to three times per week to nourish the hair. Niacin is also included in the formulation to improve circulation.

Research studies in both Finland and France showed 80 percent of those tested experienced positive results. Seventy dermatologists participated in the French study. The product was found to be safe and effective, with no side effects reported.

## SUMMING IT UP

Let's face it, male pattern baldness is genetically determined and influenced by the hormone DHT. Of course there are other factors to consider—stress, poor diet, hypothyroidism, drugs, poor circulation, parasites, etc. over which you do have some control. While massage,

* Available through Nature's Distributors 1-800-624-7114.

exercise, and use of a slant board can help circulation, nutritional changes are important.

The cells of hair follicles produce hair when they are supplied with the nutrients they need. In a balding man, the cells aren't receiving the needed nourishment and consequently the hair-producing cells die off creating a case of cellular malnutrition. The challenge is to find a way to nourish the hair cells. This cannot be accomplished with drugs—in fact, they produce an opposite effect. We can begin by nourishing the body as a whole—eliminating processed foods, choosing and balancing quality macronutrients.

Adding supplemental nutrients for the hair to your diet can also help. These nutrients should include the B vitamins (specifically biotin, PABA, pantothenic acid, and inositol), as well as vitamin E, iron, zinc, methionine and cysteine, and EFAs.

No matter which program you decide to follow, do allow up to three months before you see results. The best approach is both topical and internal. And, just to cover all bases, I usually suggest that all my hair-loss clients get an amino acid profile from Aatron (1-800-367-7744).

# CHAPTER 9

# SUPER NUTRITION
# FOR SUBSTANCE ABUSE

An amazingly effective approach to drug and alcohol rehab is one that features nutritional supplements (vitamins, minerals, amino acids, herbs), along with balanced, wholesome eating to hasten recovery. This approach, coupled with counseling, is a truly holistic one that helps to ease withdrawal symptoms and eliminate cravings. Super nutrition can work for you or a loved one, whether the addictive substance is alcohol, cigarettes, sugar, or legal or illegal drugs.

Years ago the words "substance abuse" might have conjured visions of unsavory characters shooting heroine, snorting cocaine, or smoking marijuana. Today, however, that picture has changed: Many substance abusers are clean-cut, middle-class Americans. And, it's not only illegal street drugs that are abused. FDA-approved drugs kill 140,000 people per year—seven times more than heroin, crack, and all other illegal drugs put together. **And**, the three most widely used drugs in our culture—caffeine, alcohol, and nicotine—are legal. This is not to downplay the problem we have with street drugs, but the problem doesn't stop there.

Many of my teen clients who are cocaine abusers have a similar family scenario. Dad buys and drinks booze by the case and mom routinely takes half a dozen over-the-counter and prescription drugs to calm her nerves. The **entire** family has a drug problem, not just the teen. While some drugs are no doubt more harmful than others, we need to understand that a drug is a drug is a drug. All are toxic to some degree and all rob us of vital nutrients. It is imperative that we strive to keep drug use to an absolute minimum.

In the context of this chapter I will focus primarily on alcohol and cocaine, but will touch also on cigarettes, marijuana, and coffee. You've heard repeatedly about what's wrong with these substances. I will emphasize nutritional solutions in helping to give up these substances and mitigate the discomfort of withdrawal.

Mainstream advice about kicking these habits usually consists of mustering up will power, having faith, and/or resolving emotional conflicts. While these are all desirable actions to take, they're sometimes hard to accomplish—almost impossible, in the face of a powerful, compelling addiction. I use the word "addiction" very broadly here; defined as "the experience of being unable to immediately and permanently stop the use of a drug without suffering some degree of discomfort."[1]

The missing component from most drug withdrawal programs, whether it's smoking or alcohol rehab, is biochemical repair. The addict can be counseled till the cows come home, but this won't correct the chemical imbalances (nutrient deficiencies) that perpetuate the condition. Until they are corrected, we cannot rightly claim recovery, even if abstinence from the formerly abused substance is achieved. Much of what has been called "recovery" is simply the substituting of one addiction for another. Too often detox involves getting the addict off of his drug of choice onto another drug or set of drugs. The cocaine addict who trades barbituates for tranquilizers (in the name of "treatment") isn't cured. He's just now doing a more socially acceptable drug. The alcoholic who relies on caffeine, nicotine and sugar for his highs isn't recovered. Though no longer drinking alcohol, his body chemistry remains deranged. His craving for alcohol and his mood swings and depression likely remain. **We have overcome addiction only when we are no longer dependant upon any harmful substance.**

Real recovery is about nourishing the body, freeing it from dependency upon drugs and other damaging substances, such as sugar, that can be addictive. I believe that the negative mental state that gives rise to chemical dependency is itself brought on largely by nutritional deficiency, which is further deepened by drug involvement. Drug therapy for drug addiction may mask symptoms, but it doesn't correct their cause. Replacing missing nutrients can.

## CAFFEINE

Caffeine, in the form of coffee, is the drug of choice for Americans. We consume over 400 million cups daily. Fifty percent of the population ingests at least two cups of coffee daily, 25 percent take in about five cups every day and the remaining 25 percent drink ten or more cups daily.

Caffeine is an extremely potent stimulant that is widely consumed by Americans, not only in coffee, but in teas, colas, OTC wake-up pills, diet pills, diuretics, cold remedies, headache remedies, and stimulants. It is similar in effect to amphetamines and cocaine. Chemically, caffeine is classified as a xanthine alkaloid. Other xanthines include theobromine from chocolate and theophylline from tea. All of these substances are similar in their chemical structure and their ability to stimulate the central nervous system. All three are found in coffee. Ingestion of caffeine, especially in amounts exceeding 200 mg. (about two cups of coffee), can contribute to many health problems.

The caffeine content of coffee depends upon the method used to prepare it. Coffee prepared by the drip method has the highest concentration of caffeine—about 146 mg. per cup. A cup of percolated coffee has 110 mg., while instant has 66 mgs. Even decaffeinated coffee has some caffeine, about 2-5 mg., and often traces of the chemical solvent used to remove the caffeine. The most frequently used solvent today is methylene chloride which can cause irregular or abnormal heartbeats, nausea, and vomiting. A safer, but less frequently used solvent is ethyl acetate. Coffee can also be decaffeinated by the water-process method, which is by far the most preferable. Even when caffeine is removed, however, oils, acids, tannins, and hundreds of other chemicals remain which also cause physiological changes. While the amount of caffeine in coffee ranges from 1 percent to 1.3 percent, tea leaves contain 1 percent to 5 percent, depending upon the variety, how they are processed and other factors. The standard cup of tea brewed for five minutes contains 46 mg. of caffeine. Brewed for one minute, only 28 mg. Many herbal teas contain no caffeine. Some do, however, so make sure that the label is marked "caffeine free."

Other caffeine-containing items are listed below, with the amount of caffeine indicated in mgs. Over-the-counter drugs are listed in the second column:

| | |
|---|---|
| baking chocolate—35 per oz. | Bivarin—200 per tablet |
| milk chocolate—6 per oz. | Caffedrine—200 |
| cocoa, 1 cup—13 | Aqua-ban—100 |
| Dr. Pepper—61 | Excedrin—64 |
| Mountain Dew—55 | Vanquish—33 |

Tab—49                          Anacin—32
Pepsi Cola—43                   Dristan—16
Diet RC—33                      Diet Rite—32

Health conditions with which caffeine has been linked include:

anxiety
depression
nervousness/irritability
high blood pressure
certain forms of cancer (kidney, bladder, ovary, pancreas)
heart disease/heart palpitations
ulcers
fibrocystic conditions
sleep disorders
reduced nutrient assimilation
diabetes
vision problems (glaucoma)
infertility
vitamin and mineral loss
kidney infection/failure
birth defects
adrenal exhaustion

Many men who drink coffee also smoke. Smokers need to drink a lot more coffee than non-smokers to get the same effect. Here's why: Caffeine stays in a smoker's bloodstream only half as long because the tar in cigarettes increases the rate at which enzymes metabolize it. When the ex-smoker continues to drink coffee at the same rate as when he was smoking, blood levels of caffeine increase dramatically. Tobacco withdrawal symptoms are the same as those caused by high blood levels of caffeine: Irritability, nervousness, anxiety attacks, and sleep disturbance. So, when a man stops smoking, unless he also quits drinking coffee (or greatly reduces his caffeine intake), he will not be able to rid himself of these symptoms.

Caffeine has the effect of constricting blood vessels (while alcohol dilates them). This can be an advantage to those suffering from vascular headaches, including migraines, for consuming a cup of coffee at the onset of this type of headache can help to relieve it. Because of its analgesic effect, caffeine is often added to pain medications. When a chronic coffee drinker stops, he can develop "rebound" headaches as a result of the dilating of constricted blood vessels.

Caffeine activates the sympathetic nervous system that governs the fight-or-flight reaction. It also stimulates the brain-altering hormone levels and acting on the pleasure centers, leading to repeated use. Caffeine causes the adrenal glands to secrete adrenaline that eventually leads to adrenal exhaustion. Increased heart rate, respiration, and blood pressure result. The liver responds by releasing glucose.

Just as blood sugar rises when we consume carbohydrates, it also rises when we take in caffeine—or nicotine or alcohol. This triggers the insulin response that can lead to hypoglycemia (and ultimately diabetes). It also causes the body to store fat. Therefore, in addition to balancing macronutrients, we will need to eliminate (or minimize) these substances from our diet to achieve physical and mental balance and weight loss.

## KICKING THE COFFEE HABIT

Caffeine is a stimulant (as are cocaine, marijuana, speed, and hallucinogens). Neurotransmitters are easily damaged by stimulants, as well as by tranquilizers and other chemicals. These neurotransmitters, along with electrical impulses, carry information from the brain to various parts of the body. In the face of drug damage, however, messages don't always get activated properly.

Since neurotransmitters are derived from amino acids, these constituents of protein play an important part in repairing drug damage. Tyrosine—precursor of dopamine, norepinephrine, thyroid hormones, and epinephrine (adrenaline)—has been used as an effective treatment for caffeine withdrawal and for cocaine addiction. These and other addictive drugs are thought to produce their highs by stimulating the production of dopamine. Repeated use leads to overstimulation and subsequent burnout of dopamine and other neurotransmitters. The therapeutic effect of tyrosine lies in its ability to replace vital brain chemicals. Tyrosine can be helpful in dealing with the symptoms of caffeine withdrawal. Doses of 1,000 to 2,000 mg. taken three times daily on an empty stomach about half an hour before meals can help reduce caffeine cravings. Tyrosine should not be taken, however, by those on MAO-inhibiting drugs.

Caffeine addiction damages nerve synapses. Withdrawal symptoms—tiredness, irritability, headaches, insomnia—can be averted with adequate amounts of the most common neurotransmitter, acetylcholine. This brain chemical will repair the nerve-synapse damage. It is manufactured from two substances, acetyl coenzyme A and choline, a B vitamin found in fish, liver, eggs, soybeans, peanuts, brewer's yeast, wheat germ, and lecithin. Five hundred mg. of choline taken three times daily can help ease the discomfort of caffeine withdrawal.

Dr. Bernard Green, author of *Getting Over Getting High* suggests that 2000 mg. of $B_{12}$, taken in time-release form, will provide an energy boost and all the mental acuity of a cup of coffee in the morning. It should be taken in conjunction with a high potency B vitamin tablet or a multiple vitamin/mineral that contains all of the B vitamins. Morning exercise can also help to energize the body and relieve tension.

In breaking the coffee habit, it is advisable to gradually substitute decaffeinated for regular coffee. Start with making every fourth cup decaf, then every third, etc., but do not increase the total number of cups consumed daily. Stick with your usual intake initially. Some people dilute their coffee with more water and less coffee going into each successive cup until finally they're drinking nothing but hot water. You may want to cut back by eliminating one cup every three to four days. Another option is to replace coffee (gradually) with herb teas (valerian or chamomile to relax are good) or one of the grain-base coffee substitutes, such as Pero or Roma.

Providing the nutritional support your body needs is perhaps the most important thing you can do. In addition to the B vitamins, vitamin C (1000 mg.), calcium, and magnesium can be helpful in combating stress. Vitamin C will also help detoxify the body. Extra C (1,000 mg.), along with 250 mg. of $B_6$ twice daily, will help rid the body of excess liquid which can accumulate when coffee (itself a diuretic) is stopped. This extra C and $B_6$ can be discontinued in a few days.

Another antioxidant, vitamin E, can be helpful in large doses (800 mg.) on a short-term basis to ease withdrawal symptoms. It, along with the $B_{12}$, choline, vitamin C, and extra calcium and magnesium should be used for a one-week period following the elimination of coffee from the diet, after which time the dose can be lowered or the supplements discontinued, depending upon symptoms. There is no harm in continuing these supplements, as well as tyrosine for as long as needed.

# NICOTINE

Whereas caffeine is a stimulant, nicotine (as well as alcohol) is a depressant. Like caffeine, it is a legally available, socially acceptable drug used widely in our culture. It is our third most popular drug, after coffee and alcohol, although its popularity has decreased in the last few decades.

Once upon a time it was stylish to smoke. Everyone did it—even doctors. In fact, cigarette advertisements declaring that more doctors smoked Lucky Strike than any other brand appeared in past editions of the *American Medical Association Journal!* That all changed in 1964 when the Surgeon General's report was issued confirming the health hazards of smoking including cancer, lung disease, and heart failure. The ensuing campaign against smoking has been surprisingly successful, considering the highly addictive nature of the drug. Per capita cigarette consumption dropped from 4,345 in 1963 to 2,493 in 1994. In 1966, 50 percent of the men in this country smoked. By 1988, only 30 percent did. Men may abuse drugs and alcohol three times as much as women do, but they do a better job of quitting once they decide to do so!

It was first established that smoking is physically addictive in 1942 when researchers found that smoker's cravings for cigarettes disappeared following nicotine injections. Today nicotine patches or chewing gum are used to help smokers wean themselves off of this deadly poison. Its poisonous nature is well known to farmers who use a concentrated spray version of the chemical as a powerful insecticide. Inside the body, nicotine has the effect of constricting blood vessels, which results in decreased blood flow to the skin and vital organs.

The toxins in cigarettes are known collectively as "tar." They are byproducts of the combustion of paper, tobacco, and chemicals used in processing. When inhaled into the lungs, this tar causes the air sacs (alveoli) there to lose their elasticity. Ultimately the bronchial tubes and windpipe also lose their elasticity and emphysema develops.

Perhaps the major cancer-causing chemical in cigarettes is benzo(a)pyrene. This carcinogenic chemical is also discharged from automobile exhaust and factory smoke stacks. Benzo(a)pyrene is considered by the American Cancer Society to be a prime cause of lung cancer, the number one killing cancer among men. They estimated that 75 percent of lung cancer deaths could be avoided if people stopped smoking. Smoking puts men at risk not only for lung cancer, but also for cancer of the kidneys, prostate gland, and bladder.

## SMOKING CESSATION

Anyone who has ever smoked and stopped—or tried to—will attest to the fact that it's not easy. The nicotine addiction is a compelling one. Smokers are hooked just like heroine addicts. But once again, the discomfort of withdrawal can be eased by providing the body with nutritional support.

One gram of tyrosine, morning and afternoon, can help stop smoking addiction. As with caffeine, choline, a high-potency B complex, and vitamin C can all help prevent the cravings associated with the drug. Smoking destroys vitamin C. This was demonstrated when nicotine was added to human blood and it was found that the ascorbic acid level in the blood dropped 24-31 percent. Smokers therefore have a higher need for the vitamin than non-smokers.

Vitamin E supplementation is also important for smokers (and those who are quitting the habit). The carbon monoxide in the smoke from cigarettes destroys the oxygen-carrying ability of hemoglobin in the blood.

Smokers have an increased need for vitamin A, as smoking lowers levels of the vitamin in the respiratory tract. Supplements of 25,000 I.U. for the smoker and aspiring non-smoker alike are recommended.

When giving up cigarettes, it's strongly advised that coffee be eliminated, as well. You've already seen how blood levels of caffeine increase as a result of smoking cessation, thus perpetuating nicotine withdrawal symptoms.

In *Seven Weeks to Sobriety*, author Joan Mathews Larson, Ph.D., observes that successful alcohol rehabilitation depends, in part, on kicking the cigarette habit. Relapse is more common among those who continue smoking. Most alcoholics smoke. While 25 percent of Americans are smokers, a whooping 83 percent of alcoholics smoke. Dr. Larson advises that in preparation for quitting, a target date—two weeks in the future—be selected. During that next two weeks, the smoker should avoid caffeine, junk food, and refined sugars, drink at least six glasses of water daily, exercise every day, and avoid acid-forming foods, such as red meat, organ meats, plums, prunes, and cranberries.

Other nutrients that can help with the withdrawal process include GABA, glutamine, zinc, and Nicoril capsules. Nicoril contains lobelia and other herbs that the manufacturer (Phyto-Pharmacia, Green Bay, WI) guarantees will help break the cigarette habit.

GABA (Gamma-Aminobutyric Acid) is an amino acid that has a powerful calming effect upon the brain. It will help counteract agitation and stress by altering certain neurotransmitters in the brain. Two capsules of "Calm Kids" (by Natrol) three times daily contain a desirable amount of GABA (133 mg. per tablet), as well as other calming nutrients (glycine, taurine, passion flower, vitamin C, calcium, magnesium, $B_6$).

Because they are cured with it, cigarettes are largely composed of sugar (up to 75 percent). The amino acid, glutamine, can serve as an alternative source of glucose to alleviate hypoglycemic reactions among smokers.

Smoking one pack per day of cigarettes deposits two to four mg. of cadmium in the lungs that can lead to emphysema. The body uses a lot of zinc to remove the cadmium build-up. Therefore, smokers are often zinc deficient and can benefit from an intake of 50 mg. per day for six weeks.

## MARIJUANA

Although marijuana, or cannabis sativa, is used by many to help them calm down or "mellow out," it is actually a stimulant. Because it is fat soluble, marijuana is stored in the fatty cells of the body and can affect the bloodstream and brain weeks or even months after it is inhaled. Being slow to leave the body, it can build up and cause unpredictable reactions.

The major problems associated with the use of "pot" appear to involve its effects upon the mental state. These include apathy, dullness, and lethargy. Emotions and desires become suppressed, short-term memory and learning ability impaired.

There appears to be some benefit associated with the use of organically grown marijuana. It's efficacy in treating visual disorders has been upheld in court and there is some evidence that it may possess properties that prevent cancer. However, if cannabis is not grown organically, a major cancer-causing agent, n-nitrosamines, can form when it combines with the chemicals in many fertilizers. Harm can also come from the psychoactive ingredients used to cut street pot. It is not uncommon for the pot sold on the streets to contain 4-6 percent of these ingredients. There are also some extremely potent hybrid forms of marijuana, such as sinsemilla. With 13 percent psychoactive ingredients, it can lead to hallucinations and emotional problems.

The tar content in marijuana is believed to be equivalent to that of cigarettes. Pot smoking can therefore create the same physical problems as cigarette smoking does. Additionally, smoking pot can create age lines and puffiness around the eyes and mouth. Men who smoke several joints daily on a consistent basis have decreased sperm counts. Like caffeine and nicotine, marijuana increases blood glucose levels, triggering the insulin response. The short-term problems associated with the use of this drug can be corrected simply by discontinuing its use. It is only with long-term use that recovery may be impaired.

The nerve damage caused by long-term use can be repaired through the use of choline (500 mg., 3 times daily), along with a high potency B complex formula. Vitamin C, 1 gram, is also recommended. It helps strengthen the adrenals and blood vessel walls. Heavy users can also benefit from the addition of pantothenic acid and $B_6$, 500 mg. each. Zinc is also important for those withdrawing from marijuana and those giving up cigarettes, for together with vitamin C, it can chelate cadmium, preventing its absorption.

When eliminating any stimulant from the body, the chemical, norepinephrine is a critical factor. The amino acid, phenylalanine, gives rise to tyrosine, which is a precursor to both norepinephrine and dopamine. When phenylalanine is not present in the proteins consumed, depression can result. It is wise to select phenylalanine-rich foods when withdrawing from marijuana, or any other drug. Such foods include turkey, cottage cheese, flounder, and roasted peanuts. The phenylalanine content of these foods helps suppress the appetite when small amounts are taken about a half an hour before meals.

Exercise should be part of any drug-withdrawal regimen. Physical activity that averages at least thirty minutes a day will help produce the "feel-good" endorphins.

## COCAINE

Cocaine has become increasingly popular in our culture in recent years and this is indeed unfortunate. Its effects can be a danger both to users and to non-users with whom they associate. A primary danger of the drug lies in the fact that a persons' reaction to it is totally unpredictable. One person may become ill, another temporarily psychotic, while a third may suffer a heart attack from the stimulation it provides.

Cocaine has a fascinating history. Here are a couple of interesting, little-known facts about the historical use of the drug: Up until 1914 it was actually used in soft drinks. That's right—coca cola once had real cocaine in it! **And**, Sigmund Freud was a heavy user of cocaine, as well as a major proponent of its use. He did not, however, consider it to be either safe or predictable.

While some people seem able to simply **use** cocaine, others end up abusing it. The difference between the user and the abuser appears to lie in the efficiency with which their bodies metabolize oxygen. Research indicates that users are normal metabolizers, while abusers have insufficient oxygen flow to the brain, which they seek to increase through the oxygen-like rush to the brain cells that the drug provides. The oxygen starvation that the abuser experiences causes him to feel depressed. That feeling is counteracted by the adrenal rush that cocaine produces.

Cocaine stimulates the sympathetic nervous system, mimicking the nerve reaction to an emergency situation. It blocks transmission of signals, holding them in the synaptic gap. It therefore works **between** the nerves, keeping the nervous system switched on, using the body's reserves of blood sugar and other nutrients for a "quick rush." In this way, cocaine, more than any other stimulant, creates nutritional deficiencies. The damage that the drug does to the nerve synapses will make it difficult for the user to think objectively. He may experience hallucinations, anxiety, and personality disorders. Coke also dehydrates the body, especially if used in conjunction with alcohol or cannabis.

Cocaine produces an increase in heart rate. When this occurs, oxygen consumption also increases. Pure oxygen will not, however, produce the same high, because it does not increase blood glucose levels, as coke. The effects of cocaine can vary in terms of degree and may include the following:

increased pulse and blood pressure
increased respiration
feelings of apprehension
nausea and vomiting
muscle twitching
radical mood changes
cyanosis of the skin
convulsions

respiratory failure
circulatory system failure
paralysis
loss of muscle reflexes
unconsciousness/loss of vital functions/death

Cocaine use increases the concentration of noropinephrine (or nora-drenaline) at the nerve synapse. The result is that the body is pushed into a higher state of metabolism. Consequently, more free radicals are generated. This can lead to the development of degenerative-disease conditions.

Some of the substances with which cocaine is cut—such as tetracaine, butacine, lidocaine, PCP, methedrine—can themselves be as dangerous or more so than coke itself. Withdrawal programs must be designed to offset the effects of these adulterants, as well as that of the cocaine itself.

In *Getting Off Cocaine,*[2] Michael Weiner, Ph.D., outlines a thirty-day program designed to break the addiction. I will cover highlights of his program, adding some other suggestions in the section that follows.

## COCAINE WITHDRAWAL

Weiner recommends a high-protein diet combined with specific amino acids to repair nerve synapse damage and give a natural energy boost, while taking the edge off of the agitation caused by the cocaine. These amino acids, as well as specific vitamins and minerals used in his program, are associated with brain metabolism. The program is designed to increase blood and oxygen supply to the brain, stabilize blood sugar, and provide anti-oxidant protection. It incorporates the following elements, in addition to a multiple vitamin/mineral:

| | | |
|---|---|---|
| vitamin C | phenylalanine | tryptophan |
| Vitamin E | DMG | cysteine |
| glutamine | adrenal extract | passiflora |
| vitamin B complex | lecithin | gota kola |
| calcium/magnesium | tyrosine | Sudafed |
| selenium | | |

I've already discussed the nutrients listed in the first two columns, but will briefly review them here:

Vitamin C—an important antioxidant that offsets free radical damage; plays a key role in the production of neurotransmitters in the brain; helps with anxiety, insomnia; preserves vitamin E; and supports the adrenal glands.

Vitamin E—facilitates oxygen utilization, calms the nervous system, and restores function of a damaged liver.

Tyrosine—is derived from phenylalanine; helps overcome depression, increases mental alertness, and improves memory; and is involved in the manufacture of adrenaline, noradrenaline, dopamine, and thyroid hormones. In a cocaine-detoxification program conducted at Columbia University, investigators reported that 75-80 percent of those treated with tyrosine were able to stop cocaine use completely or decrease its use by at least 50 percent.

Selenium—protects against free radicals; required to activate vitamin E.

DMG—improves oxygen utilization at the cellular level; combats fatigue; and increases endurance.

Glutamine—the only substance, other than glucose, which can serve as fuel for the brain; helps to improve intelligence, fight fatigue and depression, and control craving for sugar and alcohol.

Vitamin B complex—helps combat depression, fatigue, weakness, and stress.

Calcium/magnesium—help eliminate muscle cramping and twitching; a natural tranquilizers and muscle relaxants.

Phenylalanine—gives rise to tyrosine; creates a natural feeling of well-being; helps overcome depression; increases mental alertness; improves memory; helps suppress appetite.

Adrenal extract—combats adrenal exhaustion caused by cocaine use and characterized by low blood sugar, fatigue, lethargy, depression, irritability, inability to concentrate, weakness, and poor appetite.

Lecithin—contains choline from which the neurotransmitter acetylcholine is derived. Acetlycholine is responsible for nerve transmission; it regulates the activity of the muscles, is required for memory, appetite, sexual behavior, and the ability to sleep. Choline and lecithin can have an anti-depressant effect and help combat physical restlessness.

The third column on page 148 contains substances not previously described. The first item, tryptophan, was included in Weiner's program before the FDA prohibited its manufacture and sale in the fall of 1989, following the discovery of a contaminated batch. Prior to that time, the amino acid had been used successfully in drug and alcohol rehabilitation programs with no ill-effects. Tryptophan helps to offset depression by increasing levels of the neurotransmitter, serotonin. It has an anti-anxiety effect and helps combat insomnia. While the ban on tryptophan is in effect, one should not attempt to obtain it. Melatonin, 6 mg., can be used in its place to help induce sleep. Inositol can help, as well. It is a B vitamin found in lecithin.

Cysteine, a sulphur-containing amino acid, helps to destroy harmful chemicals in the body, such as acetylaldehyde and free radicals produced by smoking, drinking, and the body's metabolic processes. It protects against radiation, heavy metals, and other harmful substances.

Passiflora or passion flower is a sedative herb. One type of passion flower, Giant Granadilla, has been found to contain serotonin. It helps to calm the body by promoting transmission of subtle nerve impulses. It is useful to combat insomnia, nervous tension, fatigue, and muscle spasms.

Gota Kola is another herb that has sedative properties. It also is a tonic herb that can strengthen and energize the brain.

Sudafed is a synthetic version of the Chinese herb, ma haung (ephedra). It is an over-the-counter pharmaceutical used to treat allergies. The drug stimulates the central nervous system without raising blood sugar. It is similar pharmacologically to cocaine, except the stimulation from it lasts a few hours, instead of just a few minutes, as with cocaine. Weiner recommends that Sudafed be used during the first few days of withdrawal from cocaine or amphetamines. He emphasizes the importance of reading the cautions on the label and not exceeding one 30 mg. tablet twice daily. He further recommends that it not be taken more than five days without consulting a physician.

In addition to the above, Weiner emphasizes the importance of consuming foods high in phenylalanine to facilitate noradrenaline production. He also recommends that high carbohydrate meals be avoided because they will "slow you down and make you drowsy." Good advice. For hallucinations, he advises use of niacin and more vitamin C; for nasal tissue irritation, the use of aloe vera or an herbal ointment with vitamin E or golden seal.

Apart from his nutritional advice, Weiner promotes daily exercise, 15-20 minutes per day to oxygenate the system, and the use of coffee enemas to detoxify the body. The caffeine in the coffee stimulates the liver and colon. Absorbed into the portal system, coffee can help flush out the bile in the liver, lightening its toxic load. The same results are not achieved by drinking coffee, due to chemical changes that occur in the stomach. To prepare the coffee: Boil four heaping tablespoons of ground coffee in two cups of water for ten minutes. Dilute with cold water to make 1½-2 quarts. Adjust temperature as needed. Pour into enema bag.

I believe that Weiner's recommendations are excellent, though I'd advise doing without the Sudafed if possible. Herbs not mentioned by him that can help detoxify the liver and digestive tract include:

Milk thistle—effective in treating cirrhosis, chronic hepatitis, and alcohol-induced fatty liver. Protects the liver cells from damage by environmental and internal toxins.

Goldenseal—a liver and blood detoxifier and natural antibiotic, it helps reverse liver damage and treat a variety of infections.

Dandelion—increases the flow of bile; purifies the blood; specific for hypoglycemia.

Burdock root—a strong liver purifier, burdock helps to balance hormones.

Ginko biloba—can be useful in supporting the nervous system. It improves cellular glucose uptake, is a free radical scavenger, improves short term memory, and enhances energy.

In addition, the use of enzymes and acidophilus in any withdrawal program can enhance its effectiveness. Acidophilus provides "friendly" intestinal flora that help to digest food and control pathogenic yeast, bacteria, viruses, and parasites. Enzymes assist in the digestive process.

## ALCOHOL

One of the most comprehensive and sound alcohol rehabilitation programs I've encountered is that described in *Seven Weeks to Sobriety*[3] by author, Joan Mathews Larson. Dr. Larson, Director of Health Recovery Center (HRC) in Minneapolis, MN, earned her Ph.D., in part, by compiling the data in this book. It is a skillful blend of nutritional research, practical application, personal insight and a do-it-yourself rehabilitation program. Dr. Larson's personal insight was facilitated by a personal tragedy that drove her to understand the causes of alcoholism and to seek out effective treatment methods. Years before she became involved in the world of rehabilitation, Larson was suddenly widowed and left with three children. Shortly after her husband's untimely death, her middle child began exhibiting mood swings that were found to result from alcohol-induced hypoglycemia. Despite the fact that he was given the best of care and treatment over the next several years, the boy committed suicide in his senior year of high school.

Larson's search for answers led her to theorize that physical rehabilitation was the missing link in the treatment of alcoholism. To test that
theory, she founded HRC in 1981. As of 1992, when the book was
published, over three-quarters of the more than 1,000 alcoholics and
drug addicts treated there were successfully rehabilitated. This is
extremely impressive, since the typical success rate in alcohol rehab is
only 25 percent. HRC today provides a working model of a holistic
approach to rehabilitation—one that incorporates other aspects of
treatment, such as counseling, but emphasizes biochemical repair of
the damage caused by drug and alcohol-induced nutritional imbalances
and deficiencies. Much of the information that follows is based upon
Dr. Larson's compilation of research data and its application at HRC.

Alcoholism is the third leading cause of death in the U.S. Relapse is
common among alcoholics. Nearly 80 percent who receive traditional
treatment relapse within two years. Most alcoholics today do not
recover. They die prematurely from alcohol-induced disease.

Dr. Larson accurately observes that most addicts have one or more
of the following problems:

nutrient deficiency
allergies
thyroid disorders
hypoglycemia
candida

To this list we might also add heavy metal toxicity. To get someone off
of alcohol (or any other drug) and fail to treat these underlying disorders is a predictable prelude to failure. The above conditions incorporate many symptoms that masquerade as psychological problems.
Therefore, counseling is traditionally used as a primary-treatment
modality. While it can be an important adjunct therapy, counseling
alone will obviously do nothing to correct the above disorders, all root-
ed in physical imbalances.

Of those conditions listed above, I have already discussed hypothyroidism (Chapter 8) and touched upon heavy metals. There seems to be
evidence that a build-up of lead and cadmium in the body can predis-
pose one to alcohol addiction. Hypoglycemia can be caused by alcohol
consumption because alcohol triggers the insulin response. It can also
be brought on by excess consumption of sugar and caffeine and aggra-
vated by alcohol. The condition can be regulated very effectively with

the 4/30/30 eating plan. Let's now explore the remaining conditions, nutritional deficiencies, food allergies, and candida.

## NUTRITIONAL DEFICIENCIES

Detoxification is just the beginning of biochemical repair, but it is an important beginning. Listed below are the supplements utilized in Dr. Larson's detox formula, plus dose per capsule:

glutamine (500 mg.)                    calcium/magnesium(300/150 mg.)
mixed amino acids (750 mg.)            Evening Primrose oil (500 mg.)
DL-phenylalanine (500 mg.)             Multi vitamin/mineral
vitamin C (1000 mg.)                   pancreatic enzymes (425 mg.)

From previous discussion, you're familiar with each of these, except perhaps the DL form of phenylalanine. Most amino acids are used just in their L form. I've already described the effects of L-phenylalanine: I just left off the "L." By adding the D to the L form, we get the added effect of pain control and mood elevation through increased endorphin production.

In the context of Larson's seven-week program, week one is devoted to assessing the damage done by drugs or alcohol, week two to breaking the addiction. That's where the above program comes in. She actually gives two versions of this detox formula. They differ only in terms of nutrient doses. In both cases, however, multiple capsules are taken nine times daily. A person's "alcohol biotype" is what determines which version of the detox formula he will take. For details on the doses of Larson's detox formula(s) and additional nutrients used in the remaining five weeks of treatment, I refer you to her book. I will, however, give a brief overview of alcoholic biotypes (following completion of the discussion of underlying disorders), for they offer a key to understanding the nature of the disease.

## CANDIDA

Candida albicans is a yeast organism that normally populates the GI tract without causing problems. Several factors can, however, cause candida to change into its fungal form and proliferate in the GI tract and elsewhere, causing symptoms. The body systems most sensitive to the yeast are the GI and genitourinary tracts and the endocrine, nervous, and immune systems. Symptoms of candida albicans can include bloating, gas, depression, irritability, inability to concentrate, low energy levels, chemical sensitivities, allergies, and altered bowel function.

According to Dr. Larson, analysis of the medical records of 213 patients treated at HRC showed that 55 percent of the women and 35 percent of the men had case histories that indicated probable candida overgrowth.

Candida overgrowth is caused by many factors. Chief among them is perhaps antibiotic therapy. By destroying all bacteria in the GI tract, the helpful, as well as the harmful, antibiotics reduce the body's immunity and pave the way for proliferation of candida. Refined carbohydrates, steroids, coffee, fluoridated and chlorinated water, and mercury toxicity can also contribute to candida overgrowth by destroying beneficial bacteria in the intestines.

In treating candida, these substances must be avoided. Foods with a high content of yeast or molds should also be avoided. This includes alcoholic beverages, cheeses, dried fruits, and peanuts. Refined sugars should also be avoided, as well as dairy products (due to their trace levels of antibiotics) and all known allergens. Vegetables, proteins, and whole grains may be eaten freely.

## ALLERGIES

Allergies include food and chemical sensitivities. Dr. Larson states that 56 percent of the clients at HRC were found to be sensitive to chemicals in the environment. The most common allergen was ethanol, which is contained in such products as:

| | |
|---|---|
| natural gas | tobacco smoke |
| gasoline | hydrocarbons |
| certain hand lotions & perfumes | alcohols |
| soft plastics (new car odors) | automobile exhaust |

Exposure to any of these substances, as well as other chemicals, can trigger intense and sudden responses of anger or sorrow. Fatigue, exhaustion, spaciness, mental confusion, depression, cravings, and irritability can also result.

Many men have occupational exposure to chemicals. House painters, garage mechanics, hair stylists, and printers, among others, breathe in chemical fumes on the job. Those in such occupations are often alcoholic, according to Larson. They become intoxicated by the fumes from their jobs. After a day at work, they are drawn to drink alcohol to stave off withdrawal symptoms. Attempts to stop drinking can be foiled by strong cravings for alcohol.

It was the work of allergist Theron Randolph, M.D., that first made us aware of the link between environmental chemical sensitivity and many physical and emotional disorders. Special sublingual allergy testing, where a sample of the chemical is placed under the tongue can reveal chemical sensitivities. Such testing is done by a clinical ecologist/allergist who is trained not only to identify such allergies, but to desensitize patients to the offending substances.*

A biological predisposition to both chemical and food intolerances can be inherited. While clinical ecologists can also test for the food allergies that can trigger the same sort of reactions as environmental chemicals can, there are some techniques you can apply on your own to identify troublesome foods. Those most under suspicion are the foods most frequently consumed. We tend to develop adaptive addictions. Wheat, milk, and corn are common allergens for many people. One technique for identifying food allergens involves using the pulse test. Here a regular, resting pulse rate is established by taking the pulse several times throughout the day and recording it for one full minute. Once the average daily pulse has been established, take your pulse after eating a single food. Take it both five minutes after and twenty-five minutes after. A pulse 12 or more beats per minute faster or slower than your norm indicates an allergic reaction. Once an allergen has been identified, that food should be eliminated from the diet for six months to a year, then rotated back in, eaten at intervals of four to seven days, but not daily. A similar rotation of tolerated foods can help prevent formation of new allergies and control existing ones.

An important thing to understand about food allergies or intolerances is this: In order for them to occur, there must be an excess of series 2 (bad) eicosanoids present. If you'll recall, this excess is the result of consuming too many carbohydrates. Too much alcohol, caffeine and/or saturated fats will have the same effect. By adopting the 40/30/30 eating plan and eliminating caffeine and alcohol, food allergies can be prevented.

* To locate a clinical ecologist in your area, contact the American Academy of Environmental Medicine, 303-622-9755.

## ALCOHOL BIOTYPES

Dr. Larson identifies three basic alcohol biotypes. The two most common are:

Allergic/addicted alcoholic chemistry
Omega-6 EFA deficient alcoholic chemistry

The allergic/addicted alcoholic is actually allergic to alcohol. It was Dr. Theron Randolph, father of clinical ecology, who put forth this theory. His work has shown that addiction to food and alcohol can produce alternating highs and lows, depending upon whether the addictive substance is present or absent.

Randolph found that many alcoholics are allergic/addicted to the sugars, grapes, and grains from which alcohol is produced. His findings are substantiated by those of Herbert Karolus, M.D., who found that the majority of 422 alcoholics he studied were allergic to wheat or rye, the grains which form the base of many distilled liquors. The allergic reaction can effect any organ of the body and can disrupt brain chemistry, altering moods and behavior. The allergic/addicted individual will invariably become ill the first time he consumes alcohol, but with repeated consumption, the body adapts. The appeal of the alcohol lies in the body's reaction to it: As an adaptive response to the alcohol (or any other allergen), the body will produce endorphins, which create euphoric feelings. The endorphin effect is followed by the unpleasant sensations of withdrawal, which drive the individual to resume drinking. Over time, the withdrawal symptoms become more intense and last longer than the high.

Allergic/addicted individuals tend to become angry, depressed, or abusive when drinking, a result of the allergic response of their brains and central nervous systems. They also tend to be binge drinkers and are prone to having hangovers.

## THE OMEGA-6 EFA DEFICIENT ALCOHOLIC

Depression is characteristic of this biotype, depression stemming from a genetic abnormality in the way EFAs are metabolized. Normally, they are converted into specific prostaglandins, such as E1 and PGE1, which prevent depression, hyperexcitability, and convulsions.

However, with this biotype, the conversion process is defective, resulting in abnormally low levels of prostaglandin E1. This causes depression.

When a person with this type of body chemistry drinks alcohol, it activates PGE1 in the brain, which replaces the depression with a feeling of well-being. However, since the brain is hampered in its ability to make new PGE1, the supply of this prostaglandin is gradually depleted. As a result, over time, alcohol seems to lose its ability to relieve depression.

Because of its gamma-linolenic acid (GLA) content, evening primrose oil can help the brain convert EFAs to PGE1. GLA is an Omega-6 EFA. It is a vitally important nutrient for this particular biotype who can be identified not only by low EFA levels, but also by ancestry and family history. The Omega-6 EFA deficient alcoholic typically has at least one grandparent who is Welsh, Irish, Scottish, Scandinavian, or Native American. He himself will generally have a long history of depression and a close relative who was either depressed or schizophrenic. There also may be a family history of eczema, cystic fibrosis, PMS, diabetes, Irritable Bowel Syndrome, or benign breast disease. Genetic history influences tolerance to alcohol in the same way it influences food tolerances.

> People from the Mediterranean areas of Europe have been drinking alcohol for more than 7,000 years. Today, they have a very low (10 percent) susceptibility to alcoholism. Those from Northern European countries, including Ireland, Scotland, Wales, northern parts of Russia and Poland and the Scandinavian countries have been using alcohol for only 1500 years. As a result, their susceptibility to alcoholism is measurably higher (20-40 percent). Native Americans (including Eskimos) had no access to alcohol until 300 years ago. Their vulnerability to alcoholism is extraordinarily high (80-90 percent).[4]

Dr. Larson tells of a study conducted in Scotland where David Horrobin, M.D., worked with two groups of alcoholics whose EFA levels were 50 percent below normal. One group was given EFA replacement; the other a placebo. The EFA replacement group exhibited far fewer withdrawal symptoms than the placebo group and, three months later, their liver function was almost normal, while there was no significant improvement seen in the liver function of the placebo group. A year later, only 28 percent of the placebo group remained sober, while 83 percent of the EFA replacement group remained sober—and free of depression.

## HIGH POINTS

It's going to be necessary to withdraw from all addictive substances to rightfully claim recovery. People with addictive chemistries usually use multiple drugs. In that case, there's no need to employ a different program for withdrawal from each drug. All can be addressed at once with a single program. Along with this program, you may wish to use other suggestions mentioned in this chapter. The elimination of processed foods and the incorporation of a balanced eating plan (40/30/30) should be an integral part of your withdrawal and maintenance program.*

> The most commonly abused substances in our culture are caffeine, alcohol and nicotine, in that order.
>
> Traditional rehabilitation programs focus on counseling, neglecting physical rehabilitation, best accomplished through nutritional therapy, and essential to recovery. True rehabilitation involves nutrient saturation, biochemical repair and withdrawal from all drugs.
>
> In treating alcoholism, it is important to address such underlying disorders as nutrient deficiency, allergies, thyroid disorders, hypoglycemia, and candida. This is also true for treatment of drug addiction.
>
> Allergies to food and alcohol can produce addiction and numerous physical and mental symptoms.

---

* Should you require professional assistance in breaking an addiction, I suggest you contact the Huxley Institute for Biosocial Research at 1-800-847-3802. They can provide you with a list of orthomolecular MDs in your area. Orthomolecular physician specialize in a nutritional approach to treating various health disorders.

You may also wish to contact Aatron (800) 367-7744 who test for amino acid levels and will direct you to a specific formula based on your individual results.

# CHAPTER 10

# SUPER NUTRITION
# AND EXERCISE

Exercise, like eating right, can change your life. A combination of balanced eating and exercise contributes to a leaner, fitter body. If you are one of the guys who exercises regularly, then you are already reaping the awesome benefits of improved health and increased longevity. What may surprise you is just how much of an impact exercise can have in this regard. Men who exercise reduce their risk of death from all causes by 70 percent, and their risk of heart attack by 39 percent.

In addition to physical health, regular exercise has an enormous impact on mental and emotional well being. For you couch potatoes out there who spend most of the time in your head, you'll be blown away by the connection between physical fitness and improved mental performance. You all know you have good reason to make exercise an integral part of your daily regimen. The only thing left is to "just do it."

Ever heard the saying, "If you want something done, ask a busy person to do it"? Busy people **do** seem to get more accomplished, including the addition of exercise to their crowded schedules. Two-thirds of all American CEOs exercise at least three times per week, while the unemployed are among those who tend to be inactive. Presumably, an unemployed man has more time to exercise than a CEO. And while the excuses of not having the means to join a health club or spa are handy, he can always take up walking, stretching, running, or any number of other exercises that can be done at home without special equipment.

Once the tried and failed excuses of lack of time and money are eliminated, you can focus on the right type of exercise for you. Men can find clues about what type of activity they're best suited for in their metabolic rate and blood type, as well as in their personal preferences and current physical condition.

## MAKING IT PERSONAL

Basically, men who turn food into energy at a slow rate (slow burners) can benefit most from fast-paced exercise, such as running, cycling, and other aerobic activities that stimulate the metabolism. Fast burners, on the other hand, are better off with exercise that will not stress and deplete their systems, exercises such as yoga, swimming, walking, gardening.

As far as blood type is concerned, B and AB types are best suited to milder forms of exercise, for overexertion can lead to exhaustion. Men with these blood types will do well with such activities as yoga, tai chi, and stretching. Those with blood type A will also require milder forms of exercise, so as not to stress their sensitive immune systems. They would be well suited to such activities as gardening, swimming, light biking, and light weight training. The man with blood type O, on the other hand, will benefit most from vigorous exercises such as tennis, long-distance biking, and team sports. Such activities will help combat fatigue and depression.

If your blood type suggests one type of activity, but your metabolic rate suggests another, you may want to alternate, doing vigorous activities one day, and gentler ones the next.

In addition to making formal exercise part of your lifestyle, it is also advisable to look for opportunities to increase physical activity in the context of your daily routine. For example, try taking the stairs, instead of the elevator; choose a parking space a good distance from your destination; walk instead of drive if feasible; walk around the block during your lunch hour or take an exercise break instead of a coffee break to stimulate mental acuity.

Once an exercise program has been adopted, the next important step is to stick with it. Seventy per cent of those who begin exercise programs quit within one year. Proper nutrition, coupled with selection of an exercise program that is enjoyable, convenient, and appropriate to your personal needs should help sustain motivation. If you find, however, that your program is no longer satisfying or challenging to you, then modify it, change it, or replace it with another program, but do build the habit of exercise into your lifestyle, for your health's sake.

## AEROBIC AND ANAEROBIC EXERCISE

Aerobic literally means "with air." Aerobic exercise consists of activity that is vigorous enough to make you breath deeply on a consistent basis for an extended period of time. Aerobic exercise raises the heart rate and works the large muscle groups of the body. It is the best way to burn body fat because it reduces insulin levels (provided its benefits aren't negated by high-carbohydrate intake). After about twenty minutes of aerobic activity, fat is released from the cells in the form of fatty acids to be used as energy.

During aerobic exercise, the heart pumps more blood, resulting in increased red blood cell production, improved respiratory efficiency, and greater availability of glucose to the brain. While the average man has five million red blood cells in a cubic millimeter of blood, a man who is aerobically conditioned can have almost eight million. Also, his lungs can become twice as efficient as the average person. Engaging in aerobic exercise for thirty minutes four times per week will increase the brain's fuel supply. Aerobic exercise is best performed first thing in the morning, when your stores of carbohydrates are low and stored body fat can be accessed. Jogging, brisk walking, rowing, cross-country skiing, bicycling, and jumping rope are all forms of aerobic exercise. There are also structured, choreographed classes available through gymnasiums and health clubs.

In order to build the cardiovascular system, you must exercise at least 60-75 percent of your maximum heart rate. Maximum heart rate is easy to calculate: Just subtract your age from 220. If your goal is to exercise at 65 percent of your maximum heart rate, then take the maximum figure and multiply it by .65. The result is your "target heart rate." It should match your pulse rate after engaging in vigorous aerobic activity. Pulse should return to normal after three minutes of rest. Advanced aerobic training involves working out at 80 percent or more of your maximum heart rate.

If you are new to aerobic exercise, start out with only five to ten minutes of it and gradually work up to thirty minutes. As indicated previously, jogging two to three miles three to four times per week can bestow cardiovascular benefits by lowering cholesterol. If walking is your preferred exercise, start out at 60 percent of your maximum heart rate and work up to 80 percent over a two-month period. Walk at a brisk pace for about an hour three to four times per week. Walking at a pace fast enough to get your heart elevated, but comfortable enough to carry on a conversation is adequate to reduce your risk of heart disease by almost 30 percent.

Make sure to warm up by doing five to ten minutes of stretching exercises before walking or jogging. And do remember to breathe deeply in rhythm with your steps as you walk. Breathe in through the nose and out through the mouth, inhaling deeply and exhaling fully. During the exhalation phase of respiration you're ridding the body of toxic waste in the form of carbon dioxide.

You may choose to do your walking or jogging on a rebounder. These mini-trampolines provide a flexible jumping surface that minimizes the risk of injury. Due to the spring action of the rebounder, you won't lose energy on the downbounce. Just jumping up and down on the rebounder can provide a good work out and help to stimulate lymph flow, particularly if paired with deep breathing.

Dr. Phillip Maffetone, trainer/coach for professional athletes, including triathlete champions, Mark Allen and Mike Pigg, utilizes the 40/30/30 eating plan and advocates training at a relatively low heart rate. His formula is to subtract your age from 180 to obtain the high end of the range and then subtract 10 more to determine the low end. He claims that training in this manner will condition the body to use fat as fuel. Dr. Maffetone subscribes to the idea that aerobic and anaerobic training cannot both be developed at the same time. More information on his approach to fitness can be found in his book, *In Fitness and In Health.*

Anaerobic training doesn't aim at raising the heart rate, nor does it make you breath deeply for an extended period. Because it does not require sustained deep breathing, it doesn't build mental stamina in a consistent way, as aerobic exercise does. Strength training through weight lifting is the most popular form of anaerobic exercise among men. This type of exercise not only increases strength, but also endurance and bone density. It improves balance and general overall health. Men of all ages can benefit. Studies have shown that seniors aged fifty to ninety-nine not only reaped tremendous benefits from weight lifting, but enjoyed themselves while doing it. In one study, they worked out only twice a week, performing five exercises of large muscle groups, and still gained the benefits listed above—**and** they reported feeling much younger.

While weight lifting doesn't cause the body to breath deeply, coupling deep breathing with the exercise will provide added health benefit (and help prevent injury). As the weight is lifted, breathe out vigorously through the mouth; and as the weight is let down, breathe in fully through the nose.

Research suggests that getting adequate magnesium can actually double your strength from resistance training. It has also been demonstrated that potassium and magnesium aspartate can dramatically improve physical endurance. In 1968, physiologist, Bjorn Ahlborg, showed that five grains, given in divided doses to six trained athletes increased their endurance on a maximum exercise test by 50 percent! This beneficial effect is thought to result from increased regeneration of ATP, as well as improved flow of electrolyte transfer across cell membranes.

Because of the tension that builds in strength training, blood flow is impeded, rather than increased as it is in aerobics. This slows down circulation and causes blood pressure to rise. Therefore, this type of exercise is contraindicated for patients with hypertension or cardiac problems.

## THE BENEFITS

The **benefits** of exercise alone should make anyone a convert. I've listed a few of them below.

| | |
|---|---|
| increased circulation | improved appetite |
| increased oxygenation | better digestion |
| toning of the cardiovascular system | improved eliminations |
| regulation of the glandular system | enhanced immunity |
| lowered cholesterol | increased self-esteem |
| increased confidence | enhanced metabolic rate |
| lowered blood pressure | stronger bones & muscles |
| stress reduction | control of blood sugar |
| elimination of depression | levels |
| regulation of insulin production | increased flexibility |

The cardiovascular system is favorably affected by the increased circulation resulting from exercise. During physical activity, blood vessels dilate, supplying more blood to the muscles. During **vigorous** exercise, circulation to the muscles may increase as much as twenty-fold. According to fitness expert Joanie Greggains, star of the nationally syndicated TV show, "Morning Stretch" and who has sold more than eight million exercise videos:

> The heart is the strongest muscle in your body. It's about as big as your fist—and has a big job to do every minute of your life. This is one muscle you want to keep strong. The stronger it is, the more efficient it is at pumping more blood around your body and delivering more oxygen and nutrients to your muscles. This translates into more energy endurance for your physical health and well-being.

A fit heart is:

1. more efficient
2. more muscular, beats fewer times per minute at work and when you're resting
3. more powerful—pulse rate goes down, amount of blood pumped goes up
4. stronger—arteries become larger to allow for greater blood flow

Exercise increases not only vascular, but lymphatic circulation, as well. The lymphatic system is the body's pumping system designed to eliminate toxins from the cells. It is also an important part of the immune system, for lymphocytes (white blood cells that protect the body from invaders) are formed in lymph nodes and lymph fluid serves as a carrier medium for these immune cells. Lymphatic congestion or stagnation that results from inactivity, has a negative impact on the body's ability to defend itself. Since deep breathing, as well as physical activity, stimulates lymph flow, vigorous exercise can be especially effective in accelerating detoxification and building immunity in the body. This is perhaps the major reason why athletes are less prone to develop degenerative disease than others. While one out of three people in our culture will develop cancer, only one out of seven athletes will.

But with people who over-exercise it may be a different story. Dr. Kenneth Cooper, Founder and President of the Cooper Aerobics

Center in Dallas, Texas, warns that exercise can indeed be a problem if it is excessive. He began observing that professional athletes like iron man competitors and marathon runners were developing deadly cancers like melanoma and brain tumors. His friend Jim Fixx, author of *The Complete Book of Jogging*, dropped dead of a heart attack while jogging.

Dr. Cooper linked excessive exercise to excessive production of free radicals that eventually can break down or destroy the immune system. His new recommendations are to moderate exercise and add a good antioxidant supplement to fight oxidative damage by free radicals.

While strenuous exercise may be contraindicated for some men because of physical limitations, most can engage in moderate exercise and can increase its benefits by integrating deep breathing in rhythm with the exercise. Exercise can have the net effect of lowering blood pressure. Though systolic pressure (that generated as the heart muscle contracts) can climb as high as 180 or 190 during activity, the diastolic pressure shouldn't change. If it does, it is an indication of heart disease.

Exercise can also help to lower cholesterol. In men, this seems to occur largely through raising beneficial HDL levels. A study done in February 1995 involving 2,906 healthy, middle-aged, non-smoking male runners, showed that there was a gradual increase in HDL cholesterol observed with increased miles run.[1] Most of the changes were associated with distances of 7-14 miles per week. Jogging beyond that distance proved to be unnecessary and even counterproductive, due to the increased risk of injury. Using this study as a guideline, we may assume that the man who jogs two to three miles three to four times per week is favorably affecting his cholesterol levels.

A beneficial stimulation of the glandular system also results from exercise. This aids in the production of neurotransmitters. Neurotransmitters, you'll recall, are the brain chemicals that pass messages from cell to cell. Certain drugs, both prescription and non-prescription, such as those described in the previous chapter, alter the chemical balance in the body by affecting neurotransmitters. We've already seen how specific amino acids can help restore the balance. So can exercise. Like cocaine, exercise is a stimulant that increases norepinephrine levels. Unlike cocaine, however, it does not cause nervousness, but rather has a calming effect because of the influence of other neurotransmitters. Increased endorphin levels, which decrease pain and enhance pleasure, also result from exercise.

Because physical activity alters blood chemistry, it affects the mind. It influences mental performance, which reflects the balance of neurotransmitters. Mental functioning and emotional state can be adversely affected by minute changes in such neurotransmitters as norepinephrine, acetylcholine, dopamine, epinephrine, serotonin, and the endorphins. Just a few minutes of vigorous physical activity, however, can restore energy and mental alertness by stimulating norepinephrine production. Because serotonin and endorphin levels rise simultaneously, stress and depression are alleviated and nervousness does not result. So, if you find yourself "brain locked" in the midst of trying to perform a mental task or too depressed to concentrate, take time out to stimulate the mind by working the muscles. Jump rope (use an imaginary rope if you don't have a real one), do stretching exercises or run in place for five or ten minutes instead of taking a coffee break. It will provide the same mental lift, but without the subsequent let down.

Working muscles utilize more glycogen (stored glucose) than those that are inactive. Glycogen stores can become rapidly depleted, however, and the metabolic advantages of exercise quickly lost, if the system is overloaded with carbohydrates. When this occurs, the body is unable to regulate insulin production through exercise, being overruled by the insulin-stimulating effects of the carbohydrates. Therefore, to reap maximum benefits, exercise it must be complemented by balanced eating.

## BALANCED EATING FOR PEAK PERFORMANCE

When someone is in good physical condition we say that they are "fit." Fitness can be measured in terms of oxygen utilization (technically, VO2 max). Peak performance demands efficient delivery of oxygen to muscles. The rate at which that delivery is made is determined by red blood cells, their number and their viscosity (thickness or stickiness). This in turn is determined by the prostaglandins (or eicosanoids) generated from EFAs.

The prostaglandin PGE1, mentioned in the last chapter as being vital for treatment of the Omega-6 EFA deficient alcoholic, is also a key to increased athletic performance, for it reduces blood viscosity (platelet aggregation) and increases circulation of red blood cells at the capillary level, leading to increased oxygen flow to muscle cells. PGE1 derives indirectly from GLA and directly from DGLA (see chart, p. 19), both Omega-6 EFAs, found largely in evening primrose, borage, and black currant oils. Taking in sufficient GLA from these sources can therefore lead to increased delivery of oxygen to the muscles and subsequently to improved athletic performance. However, if too much red meat is eaten, an overabundance of another Omega-6 derivative, arachidonic acid, is produced that will have a vasoconstrictive effect and therefore counteract the benefits gained. We need to balance our intake of Omega-6s, Omega-3s, and saturated fats.

You'll recall that it is not just the consumption of EFAs that determines whether the body will produce series-1 (good) or series-2 (bad) eicosanoids. It is also determined by the balance of macronutrients which we consume. In Chapter 2, I spoke at length about the balanced 40/30/30 eating plan and how it can help you to lose weight and build lean muscle mass. Balanced macronutrient consumption creates eicosanoid favorable conditions where glucagon release, triggered by protein intake, mobilizes body fat. Accessing the body's fat depots for energy spares glycogen (stored in the liver and muscles), making that fuel more available to the brain, stabilizing blood sugar levels, and preserving lean muscle mass. The protein content of a balanced meal helps maintain that muscle mass and exercise helps to build it.

The typical athlete's diet, however is composed of 70 percent carbohydrate, 15 percent protein, and 15 percent fat. **And**, the carbohydrates consumed are usually the high-glycemic variety, such as pasta, bread, and potatoes. Such a diet fosters the production of "bad" eicosanoids, precludes PGE1 production, and therefore **inhibits** athletic performance by decreasing delivery of oxygen to the muscles. In addition, such a diet will produce constant hunger and decreased mental alertness, due to the insulin response and subsequent blood sugar instability it provokes. Insulin activates an enzyme known as adipose tissue lipoprotein-lipase (AT-LPL), which takes fat out of the blood and deposits it into fat cells. In this manner, insulin acts as a fat-storage hormone. Eating a diet that is balanced in macronutrient composition reduces AT-LPL activity and body fat.

The insulin-reducing benefits of aerobic exercise can be negated by eating (or drinking) a high-carbohydrate snack before working out. Under these circumstances, insulin levels will remain elevated, regardless of intensity or duration of exercise. Eaten after the work-out, the high-carbohydrate snack will cancel out the hormonal benefits that otherwise would have been produced by the exercise.

To get the effect he's looking for in such carbohydrate loading, the athlete can instead eat a balanced snack before and after work-outs. There are several companies, like Bio-Foods, Inc., that now make a

40/30/30 nutrition bar. Eating half of such a bar before exercise will assure that the body burns stored fat for energy, rather than carbohydrates and that it produces good eicosanoids. Eating the other half after exercise helps to maintain the hormonal benefits of the balanced macronutrient intake.[2] Athletes should not consume high-fiber foods, such as whole grain or apples before exercise, for these pull water from the body into the intestinal tract. This decreases performance.

Consuming too much protein in relationship to carbohydrates can actually be worse for an athlete than eating too many carbohydrates, for it can create a state of "ketosis," which causes loss of muscle mass. Imbalance in either direction creates problems.

Another benefit of balanced eating is that the higher levels of glucagon, produced by the higher percentage of protein, stimulate the production and utilization of Human Growth Hormone, which facilitates muscle growth and repair. Series-1 eicosanoids release HGH from the pituitary. On the other hand, excess carbohydrates cause elevated insulin levels that can block hormones that increase production and effectiveness of HGH. Most of the 40/30/30 bars, unlike high-carbo sports bars, contain chromium, which improves the utilization of HGH (and amino acids) in the cells.

Although the balanced bars are a wonderful aid to athletic performance, remember that it is necessary to maintain the 40/30/30 balance at **every** meal to continually reap the benefits. I'll show you how to do this in the next chapter. For now, understand that balanced eating improves athletic performance in these ways:

> elimination of hunger
> enhanced cardiovascular endurance
> elimination of fatigue
> increased muscular endurance
> increased concentration
> reduction of body fat
> increased oxygen transfer to muscle cells
> improved recovery rate

According to Bio-Foods president, Richard Lamb,

> A number of professional, world and national class athletes have changed to a more balanced diet modeled

after the Balance program with considerable success. Among them are 7 swimming medalists in Barcelona, the Subaru-Montgomery pro cycling team, U.S. Pro cycling champion, Bart Bowen, skiers, Ewa Twardokens and Robbie Huntoon; national cycling trial champion, John Stenner, and literally dozens of nationally ranked triathletes in Southern California.

One study, conducted by the Dept. of Sports Medicine at Pepperdine University at Malibu, CA,[3] tested the difference in performance between athletes consuming a diet of 60 percent carbohydrate, 20 percent protein, and 20 percent fat and those consuming the 40/30/30 balance diet. After four weeks on these two dietary regimes, runners were asked to run four consecutive 5 km. segments on a hilly course at training pace, then a final 5 km. segment to exhaustion at race pace.

The **Balance** group ran significantly faster than the high-carbohydrate group in the last race. They also ran faster in the other segments of the race (though not significantly faster from the point-of-view of statistics) and raised their HDL (good) cholesterol level by an average of 14 points, compared to the carbohydrate group. The results of this study indicate that balanced macronutrient consumption increases a competitor's reserve for the final "kick" in competition by enabling him to utilize body fat for energy and spare muscle glycogen. At the end of the study, athletes on the **Balance** program reported "better appetite satisfaction, better recovery and better overall feelings of health and well-being."

In another study, published in *Medicine and Science in Sports and Exercise*,[4] the running times of six trained athletes were compared on diets with different fat contents, 15 percent (low), 24 percent (normal), and 38 percent (high). It was found that running time to exhaustion was greatest following the high-fat diet (91.2 min., compared to 75.8 and 69.3 min. for the normal and low-fat diets respectively). Oxygen utilization was also higher on the high-fat diet (66.4 ml/kg/min. versus 59.6 and 63.7 for the low-fat and normal diets). While I don't recommend a diet that exceeds 30 percent fat, this study does dramatically demonstrate the performance benefits to be gained by adding good fat to the diet.

The reason that increasing fat in the diet increases endurance has to do with the fact that fat yields more molecules of ATP (adenosine triphosphate, the basic energy molecule of the cell) than does glucose:

Fat yields 460 molecules, compared to glucose's 36. Also, fat stores in a healthy male adult produce 100,000 kilcalories (calories) of energy, while glucose stores (glycogen) provide only about 2,000.

All of this goes to show that, used properly, nutrition can be just as important, and very possibly more important, than physical training in shaping an athlete's performance.

## DON'T OVERDO

As you can see, exercise is enormously beneficial to your physical, mental, and emotional health. Some men, however, get carried away, pushing their bodies beyond what is healthy. An excessive amount of exercise can actually create health problems. Symptoms of over-training can include elevated resting heart rate, deteriorating performance, insomnia, lethargy, loss of appetite, soreness, irritability, diarrhea, and apathy. While moderate amounts of exercise increase bone density, mineral utilization problems can result from excessive exercise.

Since electrolytes are lost through perspiration during exercise, their replacement is desirable. This is common knowledge among athletes. What's not well known is that many so-called electrolyte formulas lack the critically important trace elements and contain harmful sugar additives (that actually leach minerals from the body). Bioavailability of the minerals in such formulas is limited. Use instead a true electrolyte formula, such as Trace-Lyte, consisting of trace, as well as macro minerals, in crystalloid form, for maximum utilization.

## REVIEW

Some major points from this chapter include:

> Balanced (40/30/30) eating enhances athletic performance, while taking in too much carbohydrate before and after exercise can cancel out its benefits.

> Aerobic exercise (jogging, brisk walking, etc.) burns fat by reducing insulin levels, as long as carbohydrate

intake is not excessive. Engaging in aerobic exercise (jogging, brisk walking, etc.) for thirty minutes four times per week will improve mental performance, as well.

Benefits of anaerobic exercise can be increased by adding deep, rhythmic breathing.

Slow burners and men with type O blood can benefit most from vigorous exercise.

# CHAPTER 11

# SUPER NUTRITION AT HOME

We're on the brink of a new revolution in healthy eating. For the past several years you have been encouraged to consume a high-carbohydrate, low-fat diet for optimum health, endurance, and weight control. We now know that you can accomplish all of these goals on a diet higher in fat and lower in carbohydrates than that advocated in recent years. The key to reduction of body fat is the very same key that unlocks the door to long-lasting energy and increased stable blood sugar. That key is control of insulin levels through the right macronutrient balance.

A good rule of thumb regarding food and insulin levels: The more processed the food, the less fiber it contains, and the worse it is going to be on insulin levels. The sample meals and recipes in this chapter emphasize whole foods that are high in fiber and meals with enough protein to keep insulin's antagonist, glucagon, activated so that you can readily access fat stores. Fat loss will result, with no need to count calories.

Although I'm more interested in inspiring you to "cut the carbs and add the fat" than to follow the 40/30/30 eating plan to the "tee," I offer guidelines below for those wishing to put the plan into action. You'll also find an expanded glycemic index in this chapter to help identify those carbohydrates that are converted quickly to blood sugar in the body and therefore trigger a rapid rise in insulin secretion.

One of the major problems with the Standard American Diet is that it contains an abundance of bad fats, mostly in the artificial, hydrogenated form. These fats are hidden in many processed, prepared foods. I'll give you some tips on avoiding these, as well as limiting the **friendly** saturated fats that can turn into enemies if not balanced with vitally important EFAs and other essential nutrients.

173

## 40/30/30 MEAL CONSTRUCTION

Below you will find 3 balanced menu suggestions for breakfast, lunch, and dinner. After each group of meals I'll give you an idea of what foods can be substituted for the underlined foods without disrupting the 40/30/30 macronutrient balance of the meal.

### Breakfasts
A.  8 ounces tomato juice
    2 poached eggs
    2 slices of 7-grain <u>toast</u> (dry)
    1/2 cup low-fat cottage cheese

B.  5-egg omelette (1 whole <u>egg</u>, 4 whites)
    1 1/2 cups cooked oatmeal
    1/2 cup skim milk
    8 ounces water, decaf coffee, or tea

C.  6-egg omelette (2 whole eggs, 4 whites)
        or 1 cup low-fat cottage cheese
    2 slices of toast or 2 pancakes
    1 piece of fruit or syrup
    8 ounces water, decaf coffee, or tea

In place of 1 slice of bread, you may choose one of the following at any meal:
    3/4 cup ready-to-eat unsweetened cereal
    1/2 cup cooked cereal
    1/2 bagel, pita, or English muffin
    1 tortilla
    1/2 cup cooked pasta
    1/3 cup cooked rice
    1/3 cup cooked beans
    1 small potato (3 oz.)

In place of 1 medium egg, select one of the items below at any meal:
    1/4 cup creamed cottage cheese or ricotta
    1 ounce veal
    1 ounce ground beef
    4 ounce tofu (soybean curd)

The fruits below have approximately the same number of carbohy-drate grams, though they differ in terms of glycemic index rating, and may be used interchangeably:

| | |
|---|---|
| 1/2 banana | 1/2 grapefruit |
| 15 small grapes | 1/3 cantaloupe |
| 2 tablespoons raisins | |
| 1 small apple, peach, orange, or pear | |
| 1/2 cup orange, apple, or grapefruit juice | |

## Lunches

A.  4 ounces tempeh with lettuce and tomato
    1 whole grain hamburger bun or 1 Pita pocket
    1 piece of low-glycemic fruit or salad

B.  1 large salad (lettuce, tomatoes, cucumber, etc. with 2 tea-spoons dressing)
    2 ounces chicken, turkey, seafood, or 2/3 cup low-fat cottage cheese
    1 piece of low-glycemic fruit or a small roll
    1 large sliced apple
    Sprinkle with 1 tablespoon granola

C.  4 ounces Albacore tuna in water
    1 tablespoon canola mayonnaise
    2 rye crisp crackers
    3 cups Romaine lettuce
    2 tablespoons fat-free Italian dressing
    1 large kiwi

The low-glycemic fruits include:

| | | | |
|---|---|---|---|
| apples | oranges | pears | grapes |
| grapefruit | plums | peaches | strawberries |

Limit bananas and dried fruits.

**Dinners**

A.  6 ounces baked or broiled halibut or sole
    2 cups cooked low-glycemic vegetables
    1 cup cooked pasta or 3-4 little red potatoes
    1 large dinner salad with 1 tablespoon salad dressing

B.  5 ounces skinned chicken breast or lean beef
    1 large baked potato or 1 1/2 cups cooked pasta
    1 cup cooked low-glycemic vegetables

C.  6 ounces soy tempeh for stir fry
    1 cup broccoli or snow peas
    1 cup *zucchini or cabbage
    1/2 red or green pepper
    1 cup cooked brown rice

*Vegetables that may be substituted for one another, without affecting the carbohydrate balance of the meal include:

1/2 cup cooked green beans          1/2 medium artichoke
1/2 cup cooked asparagus            1/2 cup cooked beets
1/2 cup cooked summer squash        1/2 cup cooked greens
1 cup raw or 1/2 cup                1/2 cup cooked Brussels
    cooked carrots                      sprouts

Low-glycemic vegetables include:

| | | | |
|---|---|---|---|
| broccoli | eggplant | Brussels sprouts | cauliflower |
| asparagus | artichoke | green beans | cucumber |
| zucchini | cabbage | celery | spinach |
| lettuce | tomato | | |

Limit carrots, corn, and peas.

One tablespoon of salad dressing has the same fat value as:

1 teaspoon butter
5 large or 10 small olives
10 large or 20 small peanuts
6 whole almonds
2 whole walnuts
1 tablespoon sunflower seeds
1/8 medium avocado
2 teaspoons shredded coconut
1 tablespoon cream cheese

For a low-glycemic dinner, try the following:

4 ounces chicken or lean protein or 6 ounces fish
3 cups low glycemic vegetables
2 servings fruit (except bananas or dried fruit)

Lean proteins include:

skinned turkey           all fresh and frozen fish
skinned chicken          tuna canned in water
low-fat cottage cheese   venison
veal chops and roasts    lean pork
egg whites               beef (USDA Select or Choice grades,
                             like round, sirloin, and flank)

**Snacks**
A. 1 plain low-fat yogurt

B. 1/3 cup low-fat cottage cheese with either 1 apple, 1 orange, 1 pineapple ring, or 2 Ry-Krisp crackers

C. 1 high-protein muffin (made with soy protein or whey)

D. 1 tablespoon peanut butter on celery

## A RECIPE SAMPLER

For those of you who are into cooking—or have a wife or significant other who is—I have included a few recipes* to get you started that follow the basic 40/30/30 formula:

## STUFFED PEPPERS

*(Serves 4)*

4 large bell peppers
1/2 pound lean ground turkey, uncooked
1 cup of short grain, brown rice
1 medium onion, chopped
1/2 teaspoon cayenne pepper
1 teaspoon Italian seasonings
2 cups marinara sauce

Preheat the oven to 350 degrees F.

Cut opening in top of peppers, clean out interior. Poach peppers in boiling water or steam for 5 minutes. In a separate bowl, mix together turkey, onions, rice, seasonings, and 1 cup of marinara. Stuff each pepper with 1/4 of the mixture. Place in covered baking dish and bake for 50-60 minutes. Pour 1/4 cup marinara on each stuffed pepper before serving.

270 calories, 29 grams carbohydrate(C)
18 grams protein (P), 10 grams fat (F)

* Recipes adapted from Bio-Foods, Inc. of Santa Barbara, CA.

## VEGGIE LASAGNA

*(Serves 8)*

1 pound lasagna noodles, undercooked
2 teaspoons olive oil
2 medium onions, sliced
3 teaspoons Italian seasonings
1 pound sliced mushrooms
2 cups fresh zucchini, sliced
1 package frozen spinach, chopped and thawed
2 24-ounce tomatoes, diced
2 cups low-fat Ricotta cheese
2 cloves garlic, minced
1/4 cup grated Parmesan cheese

Preheat oven at 350 degrees F.

In a skillet, heat olive oil, add onions and mushrooms, and cook until onions are soft. Mix in 2 teaspoons seasonings and remove from pan. Set aside. Place zucchini in skillet and lightly saute. Remove and set aside. Add diced tomatoes to onions and mushrooms and simmer for 30 minutes.

In food processor or blender, whip cottage cheese until smooth. Add ricotta cheese and whip together. Add spinach, 1 teaspoon Italian seasonings, garlic, Parmesan cheese, and blend carefully.

In a baking dish, layer noodles, cheese mixture, zucchini, noodles, half the sauce, noodles, and remaining sauce. Bake for 1 hour.

Let stand for 15 minutes before serving.

240 calories per serving, 33 grams C
21 grams P, 5 grams F

## SPICY SEAFOOD CASSEROLE

*(Serves 2-4)*

2 1/2 cups cooked brown rice
3/4 cup low fat mayonnaise
1/2 cup low fat milk
1 medium onion chopped
1/4 cup chopped green pepper
1 chopped jalapeno
1 clove garlic
1 cup fresh crab meat
1 cup fresh shrimp
1 cup tomato juice
1/4 teaspoon cayenne pepper
1/8 teaspoon cumin

Preheat oven to 350 degrees.

Mix all ingredients together. Place ingredients in lightly buttered or greased 9-by-13-inch casserole dish. Bake for 1 hour. Serve with tossed greens and enjoy!

500 calories per serving, 50 grams C
39 grams P, 16 grams F

## COOL PASTA SALAD

*(Serves 4)*

3 cups cooked tricolored rotini, drained and rinsed
2 medium tomatoes, chopped
2 stalks celery, sliced
2 green onions, sliced
2 cups broccoli flowerettes, steamed (3-5 minutes)
8 ounces grilled chicken strips (or turkey)
1 cup vinaigrette dressing
1/2 teaspoon crushed basil

Combine all ingredients and chill for 2-3 hours.
Serve on romaine lettuce (or lettuce of your choice).

330 calories per serving, 37 grams C
25 grams P, 10 grams F

# THE GLYCEMIC INDEX

In Chapter 2, I gave you a partial listing of foods from the glycemic index. A more complete listing appears below.

According to the literature put out by Bio-Foods:

> The trick to using the glycemic index is knowing when your body needs long-term energy vs. a short burst for performance. Before a long workout, a food with a low glycemic index is the best choice because you receive a long, steady release of sugar into the bloodstream. This prevents fatigue and allows you to maintain a steady pace. For intense, intermittent exercise (like basketball) or to rejuvenate your muscles after a vigorous workout, select a food that is high on the glycemic index scale.

## Glycemic Index Chart

The following index I put together for my updated and revised edition of *Beyond Pritikin* (Bantam, 1996).

A. **Rapid Inducers of Insulin**
   **Glycemic Index Greater Than 100%**
   Puffed rice
   Corn Flakes
   French baguette
   Puffed Wheat
   Maltose
   Millet
   Instant white rice
   40% Bran Flakes
   Rice Krispies
   Weetabix
   Tofu ice cream substitute

   **Glycemic Index = 100% Glucose**
   Glucose
   White bread
   Whole wheat bread

### Glycemic Index Between 90-100%
Grape Nuts
Carrots
Parsnips
Muesli cereal
Shredded Wheat
Barley (whole meal)
Apricots
Corn chips

### Glycemic Index Between 80-90%
Rolled oats
Oat bran
Honey
White rice
Brown rice
Banana
White potato
Corn
Rye Whole Meal
Shortbread
Ripe mango
Ripe papaya

### Glycemic Between 70-80%
All-Bran
Kidney Beans
Wheat (coarse)
Buckwheat
Oatmeal cookies

## B. Moderate Inducers of Insulin:
### Glycemic Index Between 60-70%
Raisins
Mars candy bar
Bulgur wheat
Spaghetti (white)
Spaghetti (whole wheat)
Pinto beans
Macaroni

**Glycemic Index Between 60-70%** (continued)
Beets
Rye (Pumpernickel)
Couscous
Wheat kernels
Apple juice
Applesauce

**Glycemic Index Between 50-60%**
Peas (Frozen)
Sucrose
Potato chips
Barley (coarse)
Dried white beans
Green bananas
Lactose
Yam

**Glycemic Index Between 40-50%**
Steel Cut Oats
Grapes
Sweet potato
Rye (whole grain)
Sponge cake
Butter beans
Navy beans
Peas (dried)
Oranges
Orange juice
Bran
Lima beans

C. **Reduced Insulin Secretion:**
**Glycemic Index Between 30-40%**
Apples
Black-eyed peas
Chick-peas
Pears
Ice cream
Milk (skim)

### Glycemic Index Between 30-40% (continued)
Milk (whole)
Yogurt
Fish sticks (breaded)
Tomato soup

### Glycemic Index Between 20-30%
Lentils
Fructose
Plums
Peaches
Grapefruit
Cherries

### Glycemic Index Between 10-20%
Soybeans
Peanuts

## CUT THE BAD FATS, ADD THE GOOD

You know by now that the bad fats are those that are refined and man-made and that saturated fats from animal sources and tropical oils are not bad except when consumed in excess and in the absence of EFAs and other nutrients. Unfortunately, tropical oils (coconut and palm kernel) got a bad name as a result of a campaign launched against them in 1986 by the American Soybean Association who objected to the widespread use of these oils because of the competition that they posed. By the end of '88, many food companies, responding to consumer fears, began replacing tropical oils with hydrogenated ones. Consequently, coconut oil now accounts for only 1-1.3 percent of the U.S. food supply. This is indeed unfortunate, considering the dangers of hydrogenated oil (enumerated in Chapter 3) and the merits of coconut oil.

Contrary to popular belief, coconut oil does not raise blood cholesterol. It has a neutral effect on it. Coconut and palm kernel oil have a high percentage of Medium Chain Triglycerides (MCT). Triglycerides are the chemical forms in which fatty acids occur in vegetable oils. MCTs are easily digested, even for men who have fat malabsorption problems. They stimulate the metabolism and thereby aid in fat-burning. Another advantage of coconut oil is that it has an anti-microbial component that kills germs.

Both hydrogenated and tropical oils can withstand high temperatures without turning rancid, as most other oils do. This makes them both good choices to use in prepared foods such as chips and crackers—from the point-of-view of product shelf life. However, from the point-of-view of *human life*, hydrogenated oils are an unhealthy choice. They contain damaging trans fatty acids (the exception being hydrogenated tropical oils, as explained in Chapter 3). Although you want to avoid cooking with oils as much as possible (bake in preference to frying), consider using coconut oil when you need it. It is an exceedingly stable oil that will not turn rancid (oxidize) easily. Unlike other oils, it need not be refrigerated, for it will keep unspoiled at room temperature for as much as a year.

Olive oil is another good choice. It contains a good balance of fatty acids and is resistant to oxidation. Flax seed oil is an excellent source of Omega-3 EFAs and contains some linoleic acid, as well. Unlike coconut and olive oil, however, flax seed (as other polyunsaturated oils) will oxidize rapidly in the presence of heat, light, and oxygen.

Never cook with it and always keep it refrigerated. The other polyunsaturated oils may be used for cooking, but should always be kept refrigerated.

## LESS THAN 50 WAYS TO TRIM THE FAT

While my emphasis is on cutting carbs, not fat, I do urge you to eliminate the bad fats and minimize the saturated fats in your diet. The September 1994 edition of *Men's Health* magazine ran an article entitled, "50 Ways to Leave Your Blubber" that gave tips on how to cut fats from foods without sacrificing taste. Some of these tips are useful and worth repeating, as they can help you to reduce saturated and hydrogenated fat intake and enable you to avoid cooking foods in ways that would expose them to oxidized oils, which can cause free radical damage:

**Breakfast**
Use one instead of two pats of butter on your toast. Never use margarine.
Substitute Canadian for regular bacon. It has less than half the (saturated) fat.
Instead of frying your pancakes, get the frozen variety and pop them in the toaster.

**Lunch**
To avoid the refined oil contained in mayonnaise, either buy it at a health food store or in the specialty section of your grocery. Make sure the label says unrefined or expeller-pressed oil—OR use mustard instead.

Instead of processed mayonnaise in your water-packed tuna sandwich, add lemon, pepper, and hot sauce.

Choose "extra lean" or "reduced fat" ham (3 grams of fat) over regular ham (6 grams of fat).

If you must have cheese on your sandwich, grate a piece of Parmesan or other hard cheese, rather than using cheese slices.

Use non-fat yogurt mixed with chopped cucumbers and a squeeze of lemon over pita bread stuffed with grilled chicken or beef strips for a low-fat gyro.

## Dinner

Choose lean cuts of red meat—loin and round—rather than ribeye, which has more than twice as much fat.

Trim visible fat from meats before cooking them.

Avoid breaded meat and fish dishes. Breading soaks up cooking oil and seals in fat.

Heat skillet before adding oil. Less fat will be absorbed by the food. Cold oil will soak into the food.

Cook vegetables in a frying pan or wok with a minimum of oil. Start with a small amount and then add water, not more oil, to provide sufficient moisture.

When eating chicken, choose white meat over dark—and pass on the skin.

Use a rack when you roast meat so it doesn't stew in the fat that drips off.

Try making a meat loaf with cooked brown rice (1/3), ground turkey (1/3), and extra lean ground beef (1/3). Top with Worcestershire, barbecue sauce, or catsup.

Make oven fries, instead of "French" fries. Slice baking potatoes, sprinkle with cayenne pepper and roast until brown.

Instead of adding butter to frozen corn, mix in salsa. Add cayenne pepper to the cooking water when preparing corn-on-the-cob.

## Snacks

Choose pretzels instead of chips, but read the label and avoid those made with hydrogenated vegetable oils.

Buy nuts in their shells. They contain less fat, and you'll spend more time shelling and less time eating. Shelled nuts are also subject to rancidity, whereas those still in their shells are protected.

If you must have chips, choose those that are baked, not fried.

Make your own tortilla chips by cutting corn tortillas into wedges and baking them on a cookie sheet at 375 degrees F. until crisp. Top with salsa.

## CONVENIENCE FOODS

Convenience foods are fast foods, like TV dinners. Due to busy lifestyles, these foods have grown in popularity in recent years, with sales of frozen dinners and entrees doubling between 1982 and 1985. The introduction of the microwave oven was a boon to frozen food sales.

Prepared foods are, by and large, not balanced, nutritious selections. The average frozen-food entree contains over 50 percent fat. Convenience foods also tend to be high in salt and low in fiber. Some are better than others, however. And if you find yourself in a position where you must prepare a quick meal, you might want to select a convenience item that is, at least, balanced in macronutrient composition. The following foods conform to the 40/30/30 formula:

### TYSON HEALTHY PORTION
Herbed chicken
(43 C, 32 P, 4F)

### SWANSON'S
Swiss steak
(36C, 27P, 11F)

### CANNED SOUPS
Progresso's Beef Minestrone
(16C, 13P, 5F)

Progresso's Chicken Barley
(14C, 10P, 3F)

Progresso's Tomato Beef with Rotini
(17C, 12P, 3F)

Healthy Choices' Chunky Beef
(14C, 10P, 1F)

Campbell's Home Cookin' Beef & Pasta
(15C, 11P, 2F)

Campbell's Home Cookin' Vegetable Beef
(15C, 11P, 2F)

Chunky Vegetable Beef
(15C, 11P, 2F)

There are, no doubt, other prepared foods on the market that are balanced in macronutrients. Read labels to discover them. And, while you're reading, look at sugar and salt content and see what additives are in the food. Stay as close to all-natural ingredients as possible and do try to use convenience foods sparingly.

## IN SUMMARY

In planning a balanced, nutritious meal, both quantity and quality of macronutrients must be taken into consideration. Start with 40/30/30 and modify as individual needs dictate. Avoid processed foods as much as possible.

Emphasize low-glycemic fruits and vegetables and lean meats in constructing a balanced meal. If you must use convenience foods, choose those that are balanced in macro-nutrient composition.

Think low fat primarily when dealing with packaged and processed foods that contain harmful fats for damage control.

# CHAPTER 12

# SUPER NUTRITION
# AWAY FROM HOME

Let's face it—Fast foods are here to stay. But, knowing how to navigate through the fast-food counters is a basic survival skill of the '90s. Today's man is super mobile and eats as many as two to three meals in restaurants every day. Who has the time to deliberate or fuss over food when you're feeling rushed? You just need a basic road map to help guide you in making the wisest food selections.

The road map we're talking about here is far from complicated. It's pretty direct, leading you to balanced meals that contain a combination of protein, carbohydrates, and fat. These meals are built on staples like lean meats, fish, eggs, low fat cheese, vegetables, beans, whole grains, salads, fruit, and natural oils and butter. Fortunately, most of these foods can be found everywhere.

Yet, it can also be a challenge to make fast foods work. Convenience carries with it its own price: You can blow your whole daily allotment of calories, fat, and salt at a single fast-food meal if you don't watch what you're eating.

Americans are eating away from home more and more. In 1987, 60 percent of our food dollars were spent eating out. That figure is expected to reach 74 percent by 1996. Sales at fast-food restaurants have been increasing by 15 percent every year. Take-out food consumption rose 13 percent in the '80s, according to a Roper poll.

By avoiding certain food items and making some substitutions, you can eat healthy, balanced meals away from home

## THE BASICS

Whether we're talking fast foods or fine dining, the food selection you make can either nourish and sustain you or cause you distress. It's up to you.

One of the biggest challenges in restaurant eating is avoiding the bad-fat traps. These fats include the artery-clogging hydrogenated oils, processed oils, margarine, and fried foods. These oils, as we've discussed, should be strictly avoided due to the trans fatty acids they contain. Some of the more common foods that contain them include those fast food-biscuits, Danish pastries, chocolate-chip cookies, muffins, french fries and onion rings, processed cheese, mayo, tartar sauce, and chicken nuggets.

You'll recall that, while no one knows for certain how much trans fat the body can tolerate, many experts feel that the daily intake should not exceed two grams. The problem is that the most popular fast foods are really top heavy with those nasty trans. In fact, nutritional expert Dr. Mary Enig found an incredible "8 grams of trans fatty acids in a large order of french fries cooked in partially hydrogenated vegetable oil, 10 grams in a typical serving of fast-food, fried chicken, or fried fish, and 8 grams in 2 oz. of imitation cheese."[1] Need I say more?

Just remember that the trans fats that you're looking to avoid, as well as the saturated ones you want to minimize, may be hiding in creamy, cheesy sauces and dressings, along with plenty of salt and sugar. That's why you want to order these on the side and use them sparingly. Instead of pouring dressing over your salad, try dipping your fork in the dressing before it goes in the salad to minimize your fat intake. Or, just squeeze lemon over your salad in place of a dressing.

As a rule of thumb, choose those sauces that are wine-based over the creamed ones. Likewise, don't make a daily habit of creamed soups; opt instead for tomato, vegetable, or bean so you won't be overloading on certain fats.

You'll also want to hold the mayo. And tuna, egg, shrimp, and chicken salads, as well as cole slaw, potato and pasta salads, all of which contain mayo. At home you can use a brand such as Spectrum, which is made with non-hydrogenated oil, like canola. Think in terms of mustard or yogurt instead of commercial mayonnaise. Guacamole, hummus (chickpea paste), or salsas, cut with lemon juice, can really satisfy your taste buds and do not contain the trans-fat factors of those mayo-based dips.

## FATS OF LIFE

Since not all fats are bad guys and are actually good for you, then do choose those foods that feature healthy or essential fats. Olive oil is a good choice and readily available in most restaurants, especially Italian, Greek, and Spanish ones. Olive oil, along with vinegar, is probably the best salad dressing you can use when eating out. Always order it, as well as sauces, on the side. Use from one to two tablespoons per meal. You may drizzle a little bit on your entree, as well as on the salad.

Seafoods are a good source of the Omega-3 EFAs. You may select from a wide variety of fish and shellfish. It may be grilled, broiled, poached, or baked in wine and seasoned with garlic and onions. Some Japanese and Chinese dishes use either sesame or peanut oil for stir frying. A delicious, heart-smart choice in Mexican restaurants is guacamole, which contains beneficial monounsaturated fats. It can be used in place of sour cream or cheese as a topping.

## THE STAFF OF LIFE

When it comes to bread, muffins, crackers, and rolls, try to limit those made with refined, white flour—which will probably be an impossible feat in most fast-food establishments. By the way, this also goes for pasta, in all of its various incarnations, because even though pasta is fat-free, it is usually made from white flour, a simple carbohydrate rapidly absorbed into the bloodstream. Best bets, when possible, are whole wheat, rye, or multi-grain. And do remember that like pasta, even sourdough, which may be fat-free, is still white and refined.

## ENTER THE ENTREE

In addition to beans, tempeh, tofu, fish, and poultry for the main protein event, consider veal, beef, and even liver. Men of certain metabolic types, especially fast burners, can handle the heavier meats.

You may want to accompany your entree with a salad, but hold the croutons—they're usually made with hydrogenated oil. Steamed veggies (preferably fresh), and a potato, brown rice, or corn-on-the-cob to which a small amount of **real** butter may be added are good choices. And do ask if that's really butter on the table. Ration yourself to about one pat per meal. Side-orders of onions, chives, leeks, and garlic can be an added flavor-boosters for your meal.

For breakfast, eggs that are scrambled, poached, or boiled (hard or soft) are a good choice. If you're hankering for whole grain cereal or fruit, just make sure to have enough protein and good fats at every meal (a scoop of low-fat cottage cheese or a dab of natural peanut butter) so you don't overdo the crash and burn carbohydrates and go looking for a pick-me-up from sugar or caffeine in an hour.

## BALANCE IN THE FAST-FOOD LANE

As far as meals-to-go are concerned, it may interest you to know that the following meals provide a pretty good balance of fats, carbohydrates and protein that conform to the 40/30/30 formula:

The grilled chicken sandwich at Arby's, Dairy Queen, Hardee's, or Carl's
(33 grams C, 28 grams P, 9 grams F)

The chicken fajita pita at Jack in the Box
(31 grams C, 28 grams P, 9 grams F)

The chili (with a few low sodium crackers) at Wendy's
(29 grams C, 24 grams P, 8 grams F)

Plus, a Taco Bell tostada is 30 percent fat. A regular burger from MacDonalds is about the same, but a Big Mac with all the trimmings is more than a whopping 50 percent fat. Some other fast food items that have the more desirable 30 percent fat content include:

| | | |
|---|---|---|
| English muffin | pancakes | bean burrito |
| regular shake or malt | vegetarian pizza | low-fat salad dressing |
| broiled chicken | baked potato with sour cream | |

While broiled chicken is 30 percent fat, baked is 35 percent, and fried is 50 percent. The latest bird on the fast-food scene is the rotisserie chicken, touted as a much healthier alternative to fried because, on the rotating spit, fat drips off.

Most other fast-food items contain over 30 percent of their calories in fat. Some go **way** over the 30 percent mark. Bacon, for example, and regular salad dressing are 75 percent fat, cheesecake 70 percent. A taco salad (with shell) is 60 percent, as is fried shrimp, fried chicken wings and thighs, a bacon cheese burger, and an egg and meat croissant.

As far as beverages are concerned, you will want to avoid soft drinks, both the regular and diet varieties, as their high phosphorus content causes calcium to be leached from the body. You will likewise do well to avoid or minimize milk and milk-based drinks. Choose bottled mineral water, seltzer or fruit juices (and dilute them with 50 percent water). Keep coffee and tea to a minimum due to their caffeine content. Because coffee can cause the body to lose minerals such as calcium, potassium, iron, and zinc, it is best to avoid, or drink **between** meals if you must have it. Select herb teas, if available, but avoid commercial iced tea mixes because they're often pre-sweetened with lots of sugar or aspartame.

## SPEAK UP

Do make your special needs known to your server. Ask questions when necessary: "Do you serve butter or margarine?" or "What are the ingredients in this dish?" And again, remember to ask for the butter, salad dressing, and sauces on the side.

Don't hesitate to inquire about methods used to prepare foods and make it clear that you don't want anything that is fried. You may want to find out what kind of fresh vegetables are available and request that those you order be steamed.

Let it be known that you'd like your meal prepared with a minimum of butter or oil (and no margarine) and that you wish to avoid anything containing mayonnaise. Ask for a lean cut of meat. Don't hesitate to ask the server for his or her suggestions.

## ETHNIC CUISINE

While American-style restaurants are the most popular in this country, other favorites include Italian, Chinese, Mexican, French, and Japanese. Middle Eastern, Indian, and Thai restaurants have also become popular, as have those featuring regional cuisines, such as Cajun and Creole. You can order delicious, balanced meals in any of these restaurants.

## Italian

It's easy to overdo on the carbs in the form of pasta, beans, and garlic bread in Italian restaurants. So blissfully resign yourself to selecting just one of these delectables so you don't OD. The really good news is that you can eat from a wide array of absolutely delicious vegetables that you can't get in a lot of other restaurants like peppers, zucchini, carrots, cauliflower, and eggplant. And, you usually can get a leafy green, like spinach or escarole here as well. Sauteed with fresh garlic or onions and a drop of olive oil or chicken broth, these veggies are out of this world.

Then, of course, there's that cheese, usually mozzarella, ricotta, and provolone. Keep it to a tasty minimum. Try linguine with red clam or mussel sauce or pasta with chicken or seafood. You can even have your pesto (that sensational combination of garlic, olive oil, basil, pine nuts, and Parmesan)—and eat it too. Ask for it on the side. Don't overlook the veal dishes—marsala, piccata, or scallopini which are usually quite outstanding in the finer Italian restaurants.

Since Italian dishes can be on the oily side, learn to lemonize by ordering several lemon wedges that can help emulsify excess oil. And once again, in the never-ending quest to cut down on carbs, have your server take the bread away immediately if you know you're going to indulge in some pasta.

## Chinese

It's real simple when you go Chinese. Just find out what dishes can be made to order and request no MSG, sugar, salt, or soy sauce. You can always add your own soy sauce at the table. If the oil is anything other than peanut, sesame, or canola oil, then order your food steamed. Create combos like beef, chicken, seafood, or tofu with rice and veggies like snow peas, water chestnuts, bean sprouts, broccoli, scallions, bamboo shoots, and bok choy (Chinese cabbage).

If you go vegetarian, try Buddha's Delight, a mix of vegetables and noodles or even eggplant with garlic sauce. You can always add some tofu to these dishes or, if you're not a soy lover, the egg drop soup will add some more protein to your meal.

Lo mein dishes, cellophane noodles (rice or mung bean noodles), with some chicken, beef, shrimp, or other kinds of seafood might also be appealing. Just remember that those oyster and black bean sauces are just loaded with salt. Try the hot mustard, minced garlic, scallions, and even some Chinese Five Spice powder instead.

Have some green tea with your meal. It's an age-old antioxidant that even prevents dental caries.

Also, try eating with chop sticks. It will probably slow you down and enhance your digestion as a result.

## Mexican
Tasty Mexican soups, such as black bean and gazpacho, are a good way to start the meal, as is guacamole with lots of fresh lemon or lime juice. Most likely you will want to avoid refried beans, as they are generally made with lard. Here again, ask to be sure. Corn or flour tortillas are good grain choices, and they can be steamed instead of fried.

You may want to select such entrees as chicken fajitas and chicken or shrimp with rice. Other smart picks include bean, chicken, or seafood burritos or enchiladas, topped with salsa and just a bit of sour cream. Just don't overdo the cheese on these dishes because it is a prime source of fat. And, if you're lucky enough to find an authentic Mexican restaurant, squash blossoms, jicama, and chayote cactus are treats for the palate.

## French
Ooh-la-la. Here you can select from a wide variety of broiled, poached, and steamed foods. Anything sauteed in wine, such as a Bordelaise sauce, is bound to be a winner. The traditional French dish, fish en papillote (cooked with herbs in its own juices), is recommended, as are such dishes as roast chicken with herbs, steamed mussels, ratatouille (a vegetable casserole), bouillabaisse, and coq au vin. Poached salmon is also a tasty choice, but avoid the heavy butter or cream sauce, in this and other selections.

## Japanese
As in Chinese cuisine, these dishes tend to feature soy sauce, which should be avoided because of its high salt content. For the same reason, you will need to go light on the teriyaki sauce (a blend of soy sauce, rice wine, and sugar), which is used as a marinade for chicken and beef entrees. Similarly, miso, a fermented soybean paste, is also high in salt. Miso is used mainly as a soup base with sea vegetables.

Japanese restaurants are known for their sushi bars. Choose your sushi with care, as raw fish dishes can often be contaminated with parasites. Go for sushi made with cooked crab and shrimp, smoked salmon, and vegetables like avocado and cucumbers.

A good meal starter is tofu-based soup made with kombu or wakame seaweeds. As an entree, try noodle dishes with vegetables and chicken, an assortment of seafoods, fish liked steamed red snapper, grilled salmon or flounder and some hijiki seaweed with mushrooms and carrots. The sea vegetables featured in Japanese cuisine are a rich source of trace minerals.

### Greek/Mediterranean

Pita (pocket) bread is routinely served in these restaurants, along with two savory vegetarian dips, hummus and Babaghanoush. Hummus is a chick-pea pate and babaghanoush is eggplant pate. Both are made with sesame butter, garlic, and lemon. Cut with tzatziki (yogurt and cucumber), each can serve as a salad dressing on its own—or, just the tzatziki alone will do the honors.

You might enjoy a flavorful grain salad, known as tabbouleh, made with bulgur wheat, parsley, onion, tomatoes, olive oil, lemon, and mint. Greek salads and others that feature feta (goat) cheese are also a nutritious choice. Try a spinach pie for a satisfying taste treat. And as a main course, you may want to try shish kabob (grilled meat and vegetables), or, if you like it hot, the souvlaki, a combination of highly seasoned lamb and beef. For a side dish, choose rice-based or wheat-based pilaf. The later is known as cous cous.

### Indian

Indian cuisine features pilafs, biryanis (rice-based dishes), and dals (bean-based ones), as well as tandoori chicken and lamb, which are cooked in a clay oven that retains the moisture from the meat. Other tasty entrees include chicken or lamb korma with coriander and yogurt sauce. Curried vegetable and chicken dishes will satisfy those who like spicy foods.

The Indian dahl salad is similar to tabbouleh, made with bulgur, snow peas, and tomato with olive oil. With it you may want to munch on pappadums (lentil wafers) or chapatis and nan (garlic or onion bread). Make sure these are baked, not fried.

Indian cuisine makes liberal use of shredded coconut, coconut oil, and coconut milk. Coconut fat is a healthy saturated fat, which will do no harm as long as it is balanced with EFAs and other essential nutrients.

**Regional Dishes**
Tasty, nutritious selections in the realm of Cajun and Creole cooking include blackened redfish, shrimp or crab boil, chicken gumbo, shrimp Creole, and seafood jambalaya (minus the salt pork used for sauteing and the ham and sausage used for seasoning). Try to keep the meals simple.

## SELECTING A RESTAURANT

Aside from personal preference in terms of the type of cuisine selected, there are other factors to consider in choosing a restaurant. You may want to select one that allows you to order a la carte, so that you may control the amount of food you receive. Obviously you're looking for a restaurant with good quality food (fresh foods, prepared in a healthful manner). You'll also want a pleasant, leisurely atmosphere.

Inspect the menu before being seated if you're unsure of whether you can get what you want. And remember: If you have questions, ask. Shop around for a restaurant that is responsive to your special requests and when you've found it, patronize it regularly and recommend it to others.

## ON THE ROAD

Take advantage of the option of ordering special meals when flying on most airlines. These can be provided if they are requested at least twenty-four hours in advance of flight time.

Special meals generally include fruit plates, cold seafood plates, deli plates, vegetarian plates, diabetic plates, and low-calorie and low-cholesterol plates. There is variation between airlines, but all offer some special meals. These meals are often fresher, tastier, and healthier than the standard ones, as they are generally lower in salt, fat, and simple sugars and prepared in smaller numbers.

Try to avoid excessive alcohol consumption when flying, particularly if you're seated in the front of the plane where drinks are free. Limit yourself to a glass of wine with your meal and perhaps an after-dinner drink. Also, make sure that you drink plenty of water while flying, as dehydration can be a problem (due to moisture being withdrawn by the AC system). A good rule of thumb is to drink one glass of water for every half hour in the air. If you're taking a long flight, you may want to select an aisle seat that offers easy access to the restroom!

Cruise lines will also honor requests for special meals made twenty-four hours in advance of departure time. Perhaps the biggest challenge on a cruise is to avoid overeating, for lavish meals are served on pretty much an ongoing basis. Take advantage of the exercise facilities present on board to walk, run, or swim off the extra calories you may pack away.

When spending nights in a town away from home, look for a hotel that has exercise facilities, so that you can keep up with your fitness program. The tendency while traveling is to overeat and to do without exercise. This combination can undo all benefits you've accrued at home if you're not alert to the dangers and take steps to counter them.

## REVIEW

You can enjoy a variety of different types of cuisine while dining out and still get balanced, nutritious meals.

Even fast-food restaurants and packaged convenience foods can offer entrees that are balanced in terms of macronutrient content, though many have other problems, such as high salt content and lost nutrients resulting from processing. Avoid these whenever possible.

While traveling by air or sea, you can order special meals to assure the best available nutrition.

# AFTERWORD

Now that you're eating smarter, taking dietary supplements, and getting fit again, it only makes sense to plan for body maintenance on a routine basis.

In your twenties and thirties, have an annual medical exam. Have your doctor order a complete blood profile that measures cholesterol and HDL, as well as the special screening tests for lipoprotein(a) and iron overload (TIBC and SI). Keep a record of your test results to assess your progress.

During your forties, it's time to add that yearly PSA (Prostate Specific Antigen) and DRE (Digital Rectal Exam). Since I have seen so many men in their fifties with a prostate cancer diagnosis, it seems to me that earlier diagnosis might have prevented or controlled the situation. Remember that there are lots of alternative treatments to the more invasive conventional ones that use surgery and radiation. The practice of "watchful waiting" should be considered—and get more than one opinion.

When you hit fifty, the addition of a yearly stool test and a sigmoidoscopy every three to five years is helpful to rule out colo-rectal cancer.

If you travel or back-pack or eat out in ethnic restaurants that specialize in exotic and raw dishes (like sushi), the purged stool test from Uni-Key (1-800-888-4353) is highly recommended, regardless of your age. This is also a useful screening device to rule out parasites in unresolved cases of chronic fatigue, irritable bowel syndrome, digestive disturbances, persistent flu-like symptoms, arthritic aches and pains, and insomnia.

Now that you've got the knowledge, and the tools to put the knowledge to work in your life, it's time to do something about your health. Follow my advice, and I guarantee you results. You can become a mean, lean, fat-burning machine. And in the process feel better, look better, and enjoy it all because you're healthier.

# APPENDIX A

# SUPER NUTRITION MALE MULTIPLE

Here is an example of a daily, broad-spectrum, iron-free formula that can be used alone—for those that are just not vitamin-takers—or, in conjunction with the other formulas mentioned in the book.

| | |
|---|---|
| Vitamin A | 2,500 I.U. |
| Beta-carotene | 15,000 I.U. |
| Vitamin $B_1$ | 50 mg. |
| Vitamin $B_2$ | 50 mg. |
| Vitamin $B_3$ | 50 mg. |
| Pantothenic Acid | 50 mg. |
| Vitamin $B_6$ | 50 mg. |
| Vitamin $B_{12}$ | 800 mcg. |
| Biotin | 60 mcg. |
| Folic Acid | 400 mcg. |
| PABA | 50 mg. |
| Inositol | 50 mg. |
| Choline | 50 mg. |
| Vitamin C | 300 mg. |
| Vitamin D | 200 I.U. |
| Vitamin E | 200 I.U. |
| Vitamin K | 60 mcg. |
| Calcium | 250 mg. |
| Magnesium | 250 mg. |
| Potassium | 99 mg. |

| Manganese | 5 mg. |
|-----------|-------|
| Zinc | 25 mg. |
| Boron | 1 mg. |
| Copper | 1 mg. |
| Chromium | 200 mcg. |
| Vanadium | 50 mg. |
| Iodine | 150 mcg. |
| Molybdenum | 25 mcg. |
| Selenium | 200 mcg. |

The recommendation is to take 3 tablets daily as a supplement to a balanced diet and healthy lifestyle.

For the men in my family and for my male clients, I have created a Super Nutrition Male Multiple that is available through Uni-Key (1-800-888-4353).

# SUPER NUTRITION
# PROSTATE PROGRAM

Do consider the dietary and supplement recommendations for your specific prostate condition as mentioned in the prostate chapter.

In addition to an iron-free male multiple, the Trace-Lyte electrolytes, and 2 tablespoons of flax seed oil per day, the following nutrients should be included:

| | |
|---|---|
| Vitamin A | 5,000 I.U. |
| Vitamin B$_6$ | 5 mg. |
| Zinc | 25 mg. |
| Saw Palmetto Berry Extract | 160 mg. |
| Pygeum Africanum Extract | 10 mg. |
| Freeze-Dried Raw Bovine Prostate | 150 mg. |

One to two capsules should be taken daily, preferably at breakfast and dinner.

For the men in my family and for my male clients, I have created a Super Nutrition prostate formula available through Uni-Key (1-800-888-4353).

# APPENDIX C

# SUPER NUTRITION CARDIOVASCULAR PROGRAM

Do consider the dietary and supplement recommendations for your specific cardiovascular condition as mentioned in the heart chapter.

In addition to the iron-free multiple, the Trace-Lyte electrolytes, and 2 tablespoons of flax seed oil per day, the following nutrients should be included:

| | |
|---|---|
| Vitamin A (beta carotene) | 5,000 I.U. |
| Vitamin B$_3$ (niacin) | 100 mg. |
| Inositol | 250 mg. |
| Choline | 250 mg. |
| Vitamin C | 1000 mg. |
| Vitamin E | 200 I.U. |
| Magnesium | 200 mg. |
| Potassium | 99 mg. |
| Hawthorne Berry | 150 mg. |

One to two tablets should be taken daily, preferably with breakfast and dinner.

For the men in my family and for my male clients, I have created a Super Nutrition cardiovascular formula available through Uni-Key (1-800-888-4353).

Do consider the dietary and supplement recommendations for your particular sexual needs as mentioned in the sex chapter.

## APPENDIX D

# SUPER NUTRITION
# SEX FORMULA

In addition to the iron-free multiple, the Trace-Lyte electrolytes, and 2 taplesoons of flax seed oil per day, the following nutrients should be include:

| | |
|---|---|
| Yohimbine | 50 mg. |
| Panax ginseng extract | 40 mg. |
| Gingko biloba leaves extract | 20 mg. |
| Saw palmetto berry extract | 40 mg. |
| Freeze-dried raw orchic tissue | 100 mg. |
| DMG | 90 mg. |

One to two capsules should be taken daily, preferably with breakfast and dinner.

For the men in my family and for my male clients, I have created a Super Nutrition sex formula available through Uni-Key (1-800-888-4353).

# NOTES

### CHAPTER 2

1. August, Lynne, M.D. "Food and Hormones." *Townsend Letter for Doctors.* April 1995, p. 56.

2. "She's Lost Weight Eating More and Exercising Less: What's the Secret?" *San Diego Union-Tribune.* August 21, 1994.

3. Walter, Hal. "Too Many Carbs!" *Body Talk.* September 1994, p. 16.

4. Crayhon, Robert. *Robert Crayhon's Nutrition Made Simple.* New York: M. Evans and Co., Inc., 1994.

### CHAPTER 3

1. Schroeder, Henry A., M.D. *The Trace Elements and Man.* Old Greenwich, Connecticut: The Devin-üdair Company, 1973, p. 152.

### CHAPTER 4

1. Murray, Michael T., N.D. *The Healing Power of Foods.* Rocklin, CA: Prima Publishing, 1993, p. 35.

2. Martlew, Gillian, N.D. *Electrolytes: The Spark of Life.* Murdock, FL: Nature's Publishing, Ltd., 1994, p. 50.

### CHAPTER 5

1. Whitaker, Julian, M.D. *Health and Healing.* Vol. 2, No. 3 (March 1992), p.1.

2. Oppenheim, Michael, M.D. *The Man's Health Book.* Englewood Cliffs, NJ: Prentice Hall, 1994.

3. Champault G., Patel, J. C., and Bonnard, A. M. "A Double Blind Trial of an Extract of the Plant Serenoa Repens in Benign Prostatic Hyperplasia." *British Journal of Clinical Pharmacology.* 18: 461-2, 1984.

4. Murray, Michael, N.D. *The Healing Power of Foods.* Rocklin, CA: Prima Publishing, p. 333.

5. Webber, M. M. "Selenium prevents the growth stimulatory effects of cadmium on human prostatic epithelium." *BioChem. Biophy Res. Commun.* 127(3): 871-77, 1985.

6. Dumrau, F. "Benign prostatic hyperplasia: Amino acid therapy for symptomatic relief." *Am J. Ger.* 10: 426-30, 1962.

7. Phillips, Robert H., Ph.D. *Coping with Prostate Cancer.* Garden City Park, NY: Avery Publishing Group. 1994. p. 186.

8. Wigle, D. T., et al. "Mortality study of Canadian male farm operators: Non-Hodgkin's Lymphoma mortality and agricultural practices in Saskatchewan." *Journal of National Cancer Institute.* 82: 575-82.

9. Webber, M. M. "Effects of zinc and cadmium on the growth of human prostatic epithelium in vitro." *Nutr. Res.* 6: 35.30, 1986.

10. Reichman, Marsha E., et.al. "Serum vitamin A and subsequent development of prostate cancer in the First National Health and Nutrition Examination Survey Epidemiologic Follow-up Study." *Cancer Research.* April 15, 1990; 50: 2311-2315.

CHAPTER 6
1. West, Dr. Bruce. *Health Alert* (newsletter). Vol. 12, #2. Feb., 1995. p. 3

2. Welles, William F., D.C. *The Shocking Truth About Cholesterol.* William F. Welles, D.C. USA. 1990. p. 41.

3. Taylor, C.B., et.al. "Spontaneously Occuring Angiotoxic Derivatives of Cholesterol." *American Journal of Clinical Nutrition.* 1979, 32: 40-42.

4. MacRae, Holden S-H, PhD. "Effects of Low and High Carbohydrate Supplemented Diets on Running Performance." *Sports Medicine Training & Rehabilitation.* Vol. 4, #4, 1993, p. 322.

5. Yudkin, J. "Dietary Fat & Dietary Sugar in Relation to Ischemic Heart Disease and Diabetes." *Lancet.* 1964. 2: 4.

6. *Lancet,* Vol. 94(343): 1454-59.

7. Salonen, J. "High Stored Iron Levels Are Associated with Excess Risk of Myocardial Infarction in Eastern Finnish Men," *Circulation,* 86 (3), pp.803-811 (September 1992).

8. West, Bruce, D.C. *Health Alert* (newsletter). Vol 12, Issue 3. March 1995. p.4.

9. Ibid. p. 5.

10. Whitaker, Julian, M.D. "Congestive Heart Failure: A New Epidemic." *Health and Healing* (newsletter). Vol. 5, #4. April, 1995. p.2.

11. Azuma, J., et al. "Double-blind Randominzed Crossover Trial of Taurine in Congestive Heart Failure." *Current Therapeu. Res.* 34(4): 543-57. 1983.

12. Webster, P. O., Dyckner, T. "Intracellular Electrolytes in Cardiac Failure." *Acta Med Scand.* 707: 33-36. 1986.

13. Mindell, Earl. *Earl Mindell's Joy of Health* (newsletter). Vol. 3, #4. April 1995. pp. 2-3.

CHAPTER 7
1. Wei, Ming, et al. "Total Cholesterol and High Density Lipoprotein Cholesterol as Important Predictors of Erectile Dysfunction." *American Journal of Epidemiology.* 1994; 140: 930-7.

2. Douglass, William Campbell, M.D. "A Neglected Hormone-- Testosterone for Men and Women-- Part II". *Dr. William Campbell Douglass' Second Opinion* (newsletter). Vol. V, #4, April 1995, p. 2.

3. Walker, Dr. Morton. *Sexual Nutrition.* Avery Publishing Group: Garden City Park, NY. 1994, p. 104.

4. Ibid. p. 62.

5. Costa, M., et. al. "L-Carnitine in Idiopathic Asthenozoospermia: A Multicenter Study." *Andrologia.* 1994; 26: 155-159.

6. Walker, op. cit. 92.

7. Ibid. p. 110.

CHAPTER 8
1. Walker, Dr. Morton. "A Hair Raising Tale." *Explore More!* Number 8, 1994, p. 44.

2. Oppenheim, Michael, M.D. *The Man's Health Book.* Prentice-Hall, Inc: Englewood Cliffs, NJ. 1994, p. 190.

CHAPTER 9
1. Green, Bernard, Ph.D. *Getting Over Getting High.* Quill, New York. 1985. p. 19.

2. Weiner, Michael, Ph.D. *Getting off Cocaine.* Avon: New York, New York. 1983.

3. Larson, Joan Mathews, Ph.D. *Seven Weeks to Sobriety.* Fawcett Columbine: New York. 1992.

4. Ibid. pp. 72-3.

CHAPTER 10
1. Kokkinos, Peter, F., Ph.D., et al. "Miles Run Per Week and High-Density Lipoprotein Cholesterol Levels in Healthy, Middle-Aged Men: A Dose-Response Relationship." *Archives of Internal Medicine.* February 27, 1995; 155: 415-420.

2. Bio-Foods, Inc., Santa Barbara, CA, promotional literature

3. MacRae, Holden S-H, PhD. "Effects of Low and High Carbohydrate Supplemented Diets on Running Performance." *Sports Medicine Training & Rehabilitation.* Vol. 4, #4, 1993, p. 322.

4. Muois, et al. "Effect of Dietary Fat on Metabolic Adjustments to Maximal VO2 and Endurance on Running." *Medicine and Science in Sports & Exercise.* Vol. 4, #2, July 1993.

CHAPTER 12
1. "Now What? U.S. Study Says Margarine May be Harmful". *New York Times.* October 7, 1992, p. 1.